Aids to Paediatrics

Aids to Paediatrics

Aids to Paediatrics

Alex Habel
MB, ChB, MRCP(UK)

Consultant Paediatrician,
West Middlesex University Hospital

SECOND EDITION

CHURCHILL LIVINGSTONE
EDINBURGH LONDON MELBOURNE AND NEW YORK 1988

CHURCHILL LIVINGSTONE
Medical Division of Longman Group UK Limited

Distributed in the United States of America by
Churchill Livingstone Inc., 1560 Broadway, New
York, N.Y. 10036, and by associated companies,
branches and representatives throughout the
world.

First published 1982
Second Edition 1988

ISBN 0-443-03443-5

British Library Cataloguing in Publication Data
Habel, Alex
   Aids to paediatrics. — 2nd ed.
   1. Paediatrics
   I. Title
   618.92   RJ45

Library of Congress Cataloging in Publication Data
Habel, Alex.
   Aids to paediatrics.
   Includes index.
   1. Pediatrics — Outlines, syllabi, etc. I. Title.
[DNLM: 1. Pediatrics — outlines. WS 18 H113a]
RJ48.3.H33 1988   618.92   87–23853
ISBN 0-443-03443-5

Produced by Longman Singapore Publishers (Pte) Ltd.
Printed in Singapore.

Preface

Despite many excellent textbooks, the Aids series continues to fill a need. In this format the wood can be seen for the trees, essential in both clinical practice and examinations.

Aids to Paediatrics has been written primarily for postgraduate students. Normal variations and differences from adults in clinical examination and laboratory investigations introduce most chapters. Causes are tabulated with special emphasis on the relation of age to the condition or system involved.

Causes are given in order of frequency and/or importance, and advantage can be made of this fact if the lists seem excessively long. They have been compiled from standard texts, some of which are mentioned below, and are comprehensive, but not exhaustive.

For this second edition new sections have been included on Behaviour, Applying for Jobs and Preparation for the Membership Examination, and all chapters have been brought thoroughly up to date with a particular emphasis on clinical aspects.

To aid quick revision selected references for special topics are given, and have been chosen for conciseness or useful explanation. Recommendation of the most popular books for the day was thought to be more useful for a book like this than a long bibliography.

For rapid perusal, use Rendle-Short, Gray and Dodge (1985) *A Synopis of Children's Diseases* (6th edn, Wright) or *Essential Paediatrics* (1987) by David Hull and Derek Johnston (2nd edn, Churchill Livingstone). A problem oriented approach is used in *Hospital Paediatrics* (1984), also by D. Hull and D. I. Johnston (Churchill Livingstone), while an exam orientation is provided in *Child Health — a Textbook for the DCH* (1985) by David Harvey and Ilya Kovar (Churchill Livingstone). A good general reference is *Textbook of Paediatrics* (1984) by J. O. Forfar and G. C. Arneil (Churchill Livingstone).

Isleworth, 1988   A.H.

Acknowledgements

Thanks are due to my colleague, Dr Peter Husband, for suggesting improvements; to my wife and Ruth, Sheva, Gideon and Rafi for their forbearance; and to my colleagues who tolerate plagiarism as the sincerest form of flattery.

Acknowledgement is made for permission to reproduce Figures 13, 14, 15 and 16 from *Care of the Critically Ill Child* (1971) by R. S. Jones and J. B. Owen-Thomas (Arnold), and Figures 19 and 20 from *Understanding ECGs in Infants and Children* (1979) by L. C. Harris and E. Feinstein (Little, Brown).

Contents

Contents

Congenital abnormalities

CAUSES OF CONGENITAL ABNORMALITIES

1. Unknown
2. Genetic
3. Chromosomes
4. Maternal
   (i) Drugs
      a. Proven: thalidomide, norethisterone, antimetabolites
      b. Probable: alcohol, anticonvulsants, warfarin, anaesthetics
      c. Possible: LSD, sex hormones
   (ii) Infection: cytomegalovirus, rubella, toxoplasmosis
   (iii) Metabolic: diabetes mellitus, phenylketonuria
   (iv) Exposure: radiation, mercury
   (v) Deficiency: folic acid (?) in neural tube defects
5. Uterine
   (i) Moulding e.g. talipes, dislocation of hips
   (ii) Amniotic bands e.g. amputations, facial clefts

INCIDENCE OF CONGENITAL MALFORMATIONS

Major congenital malformations occur in 1 in 50 of all live births.
   Minor malformations occur in 1 in 25 of all live births.
Association of two or more major malformations occurs in 1 in 10 affected infants. Therefore look carefully for abnormalities in other systems if one organ/system is affected.

FETAL DEVELOPMENT AND MALFORMING (TERATOGENIC) AGENTS

Age/stage of development	Teratogens and their effects
0–3 weeks old/early embryo	Chromosomal abnormality or abortion likely from irradiation and antimetabolites
4–9 weeks old/stage of organogenesis	Abortion. Major malformation e.g. thalidomide; phocomelia; alcohol (fetal alcohol syndrome); infection (toxoplasmosis, cytomegalovirus (CMV), rubella)
10–40 weeks' fetal growth	Altered growth and organ injury, growth failure e.g. stilboestrol: vaginal carcinoma; CMV: encephalitis, pneumonia, hepatosplenomegaly

CLINICAL FEATURES OF CONGENITAL INFECTION* WITH RUBELLA, TOXOPLASMOSIS AND CYTOMEGALOVIRUS (CMV)

Clinical features	Rubella	Toxoplasmosis	CMV
Growth retardation	+	+	+
Acute encephalitis, hepatitis	+	+	+
Microcephaly, mental retardation	+	+	+
Cerebral calcification	–	+	+
Deafness	+	–	+
Retinopathy	+	+	–
Cataract	+		+
Glaucoma	+		
Stenotic pulmonary arterioles, patent ductus arteriosus	+		

* These infections are indistinguishable, in the acute phase, from disseminated herpes simplex or congenital syphilis. IgM specific antibody, viral isolation and treponema pallidum inhibition tests are indicated.

MODES OF INHERITANCE

Autosomal dominant: recurrence risk 1 in 2 if:
1. One parent has the disease e.g. adult polycystic kidney, spherocytosis, Huntington's chorea, dystrophia myotonica
2. Neither parent affected i.e. spontaneous mutation, is common, and the risk to the affected child's offspring is 1 in 2, e.g. achondroplastic child with normal parents

3. Grandparent and grandchild affected — 'skipped generation' —
   i.e. parent appears normal or is slightly affected, e.g. von
   Recklinghausen's disease; or detected only by special
   investigation e.g. a computerised tomogram of the brain
   showing characteristic calcification in tuberous sclerosis

RISK OF RECURRENCE

Autosomal recessive
One in 4. Each parent carries a single abnormal gene for a disease
found only when present in a double dose, and is thus more likely
in consanguinous unions. Examples: sickle cell disease,
thalassaemia, cystic fibrosis, infantile polycystic kidney, inborn
errors of metabolism, Werdnig-Hoffman's disease.

Sex linked (usually recessive)
Risk to boys is 1 in 2. A condition carried on the X chromosome,
which males show as they have only one in each cell. Female
carriers appear relatively or completely normal unless only one X is
present, as in Turner's syndrome (XO). Lyon's hypothesis is that
only one X chromosome is active in each cell, and the number of
'active' abnormal X's a carrier has determines whether she shows
any signs of the disease.
Mother carrier: 1 in 2 boys affected
                 1 in 2 girls carriers
Father affected: all boys normal
                 all girls carriers

Examples
1. Colour blindness
2. Glucose-6-phosphate dehydrogenase deficiency (p. 128)
3. Haemophilia A and B
4. Duchênne muscular dystrophy
5. Familial fragile X syndrome in XY males (X linked mental
   retardation)
   Frequency: 1 in 1000 males,
   Recurrence risk: 1 in 2 for boys, carrier females may be mentally
   slow
   Clinical: educationally subnormal, large ears and heads, large
   testes in adults (10% of the educationally subnormal males)
Rare but noteworthy: Lesch-Nyhan syndrome (p. 154); immunodeficiencies e.g. agammaglobulinaemia, severe combined immune-
deficiency (SCID), Wiscott-Aldrich syndrome (p. 133). Dominantly
inherited sex-linked diseases, in which the female carrier is often
affected, include nephrogenic diabetes insipidus, vitamin D
resistant rickets.

MULTIFACTORIAL INHERITANCE

Interaction of an individual's genes with the environment. The likelihood of recurrence (risk) increases as the number of affected family members increases, at a rate peculiar to that condition e.g. spina bifida (vitamin/folic acid lack in genetically susceptible individuals?), recurrence risk for parents:
  risk for the general population = <1 per 1000
  risk of another after 1 affected child = 1 in 20
  risk after 2 affected children = 1 in 8

'HIGH' AND 'LOW' RISK IN GENETIC COUNSELLING

For the purpose of counselling, geneticists suggest that a recurrence rate of more than 1 in 10 is a high risk e.g. autosomal dominant, recessive, and X linked disease. A low risk is less than 1 in 10 e.g. insulin dependent diabetes (about 1 in 10 to 1 in 20 in brothers, sisters and offspring of the affected person).
  The example of multifactorial inheritance, spina bifida, shows how a family's category of risk can change.

INCIDENCE OF INHERITED DISEASE AS A PERCENTAGE OF LIVE BIRTHS

1. Chromosomes   0.6%   Abnormal number or arrangement
2. Single gene disorder   2%   Autosomal dominant, recessive and sex linked disease
3. Multifactorial   30%
   (i) Disorders often manifest at birth
       Congenital malformations = 2%, include:
          0.6% (or 6 per 1000) congenital heart disease
          0.1% (or 1 per 1000) club foot, cleft lip and palate, congenital dislocation of the hip
       N.B. the incidence of neural tube defects has been falling steadily in the UK, to about 0.4 per 1000
   (ii) Disorders becoming evident as the child develops e.g. non-specific mental retardation = 2%
   (iii) Disorders beginning in childhood e.g. atopic disease (asthma, eczema, hay fever) = 20%; migraine = 10–15%
   (iv) Disorders generally confined to childhood e.g. febrile convulsions
   (v) Disorders that may be influenced by diet, environment, stress e.g. coronary artery disease, hypertension

COMMON CAUSES OF CHROMOSOMAL DISORDERS

1. Non-disjunction of a germ cell's chromosomes at meiosis e.g. Down's syndrome (95% have 47 chromosomes), trisomies 18, 13, XXY, XXX etc.
2. Translocation of an extra chromosome or chromosomal material on to another chromosome e.g. Down's syndrome with 46 chromosomes arising spontaneously or inherited from a 45 chromosome balanced translocation carrying parent.
3. Mosaicism when at least two cell lines are present, one normal and one trisomic e.g. XX/XXX or monosomic XX/XO. A mosaic parent may pass on the abnormal number of chromosomes e.g. Down's syndrome.
4. Deletions
   (i) A whole chromosome e.g. XO Turner's syndrome
   (ii) Part of a chromosome e.g. No. 5 cri du chat syndrome (parental translocation in 15%), No. 18

Newborn

SOME NORMAL PHYSIOLOGICAL FINDINGS IN THE NEWBORN

1. *Urine*. 95% micturate within 24 hours. Delay suggests renal tract outlet obstruction, renal dysgenesis, shock. Concentrating ability (expressed as osmolality) is limited, to about 600 mosmol/kg water, twice the plasma osmolality of 300 mosmol/kg water
2. *Meconium*. 95% of healthy term infants pass meconium within 48 hours. Delay suggests organic obstruction, meconium ileus (cystic fibrosis?) or Hirschsprung's disease. Prematurity, asphyxia and drugs also cause delay (p. 24)
3. *Weight*. Loss of 5% of body weight is normal, regained by the 10th day of life. Reduced intake, infection, pyrexia, increased losses via urine, stool or skin may cause or contribute to excessive weight loss. Very low birth weight infants may lose up to 15% of body weight
4. *Respirations*. 30–50 per minute, mainly periodic
5. *Heart rate*. 120–160 beats per minute
6. *Blood pressure*. 75/50 mmHg, lower in premature infants
7. *Heart murmurs*. Soft and vibratory systolic, common in the first day, may be of limited significance, and absence of a murmur does not exclude a serious heart anomaly, where expected e.g. Down's syndrome, or presenting as respiratory distress
8. *Blood sugar:* term infant   1.6 mmol/l
                premature   1.1 mmol/l   *in the first 72 hours*
                thereafter   2.2 mmol/l
Many now prefer to maintain the blood sugar above this last level, from birth
9. *Temperature*. 37°C, maintained by brown fat and environmental heat. Remember the 'neutral thermal environment' as that in which the baby expends least energy to maintain normal body temperature; the surrounding temperature required is inversely related to weight, gestational age and postnatal age

DEFINITIONS AND MORTALITY RATES FOR 1985 IN ENGLAND AND WALES

Stillbirth: No sign of life immediately after expulsion from mother after the 28th week of gestation. Rate 5.5 per thousand total live and stillbirths

Perinatal mortality: Number of stillbirths and deaths in the first week. Rate 9.8 per thousand total live *and* stillbirths

Neonatal mortality: Number of deaths in the first 28 days of life. Rate 5.4 per thousand *live* births

Infant mortality: Number of deaths in the first year. Rate 9.4 per thousand live births

Premature: Less than 37 weeks' completed gestation

Small for dates (SFD): Below 10th centile for length, weight and or head circumference

Postmature: 42 or more weeks' completed gestation

MAJOR CAUSES OF NEONATAL MORTALITY

1. Respiratory distress syndrome ⎰
2. Immaturity   ⎱ Prematurity (65%)
3. Asphyxia, birth injury
4. Congenital abnormalities
5. Infection

APGAR SCORE AND RELATION TO OUTCOME

	0	1 point	2 points
Appearance	White	Blue	Pink
Pulse	0	<100/min	>100/min
Grimace to clearing airways	0	Grimace	Cough, sneeze
Activity	0	Spontaneous flexion	Active
Respiratory effort	0	Irregular gasps	Regular, cries

Score: assessed at 1 and 5 minutes

Prognosis according to *US Collaborative Perinatal Project* for long-term handicap (H) in survivors, or dying in the neonatal period (D):

0–3 at 1 minute = severe asphyxia: give bag and
Mask/intubation, +/− cardiac massage   2% H, 18% D
5 minutes = risk of cerebral injury   5% H, 44% D
>10 minutes = cerebral injury and death   20% H, 80% D

4–6 at 1 minute = mild to moderate asphyxia: give
stimulation, facial oxygen   <1% H, 4 D

7–10 at 1 minute = no significant asphyxia

N.B. (i) Prognosis is independent of birth weight
     (ii) Initially satisfactory Apgar score is no guarantee of an
           uneventful perinatal period!
    (iii) Three quarters of children with cerebral plasy have 5
           minute Apgar scores of >6
     (iv) Despite Apgar score 0–3 for 10 minutes, 80% of survivors
           are normal

FETAL BLOOD GASES

Normal: pH 7.35
         pO_2 2.4–4.7 kPa (18–35 mm Hg)
         pCO_2 5.7 kPa (43 mm Hg)
Intrapartum asphyxia likely: pH Less than 7.20

A SCHEME FOR EXAMINING THE NEWBORN — 'TOP TO TOE'

Aim
To detect:
1. Congenital abnormalities, especially of limbs, hips, heart,
   abdomen and eyes
2. Transition to effective normal respiration
3. The effects of delivery and gestation on the infant
4. The presence of infection or disease

Method
1. Progress from head to feet, turn over to look at the back, look
   for midline abnormalities, compare the 2 sides of the body
2. (i) Scrutinise the face and body for characteristics e.g. of
         Down's syndrome
    (ii) Colour:
          pallor = anaemia/shock/infection
          cyanosis = central/peripheral/traumatic (p. 92)
          jaundice = visible if > 100 μmol/1 serum bilirubin. Normal
                      in 15% of newborn infants. Age, maturity and
                      severity determine action
          red = high packed cell volume e.g. small for dates, fetal
                transfusion, infant of diabetic mother
3. *Head*
   Measure occipitofrontal circumference with a paper or
   fibreglass tape, not cloth, tightly round maximum
   circumference = occiput to brow 1 cm above nasal bridge.
   Look for caput or cephalhaematoma. Feel anterior fontanelle
   for increased tension due to crying or raised intracranial
   pressure, or overriding of sutures from the birth, dehydration
   or brain not growing.

(i)   Face: birth marks, e.g. 'stork mark' normal, port wine stain abnormal; check each nostril for patency by occluding each nostril in turn with the mouth closed and seeing that the infant can draw breath. If in doubt pass a nasogastric tube.

(ii) Eyes: slight discharge common; if profuse, persistent or purulent needs evaluation. Sit baby up to examine pupils for colobomata, eyes for glaucoma, and with the ophthalmoscope on +10 lens at 10 cm elicit the red reflex (the retinal reflection) and look for dark spots or absent reflex due to presence of cataract(s)

(iii) Mouth: palate often has midline white 'dots', which are epithelial cells and called Epstein's pearls; clefts start from the uvula unless a hare lip is also present. Cleft palate may accompany a small jaw in the Pierre Robin syndrome

(iv) Ears: low position in renal problems, simple shape in Down's syndrome, note sinuses, accessory auricles, earhole patency

(v)   Neck: look for sinuses, feel for sternomastoid 'tumour' in lower third (though it is not usually felt in the first week), swelling over clavicle due to its being fractured, and thyroid enlargement-all abnormal (Fig. 22, p. 109)

4. *Upper limbs*
Symmetry, full extension, normal shape and number of digits

5. *Chest*
(i)   Observe colour, respiratory rate and effort and symmetry of chest movement.
Asymmetry suggests pneumothorax, lung collapse or compression by a diaphragmatic hernia or lobar emphysema. Observation of abdominal movements is valuable as babies rely mainly on the diaphragm; a see-saw motion of chest 'down' — abdomen 'up' on inspiration indicates severe lung collapse, as in respiratory distress syndrome (RDS), or weak intercostal muscles. The anterior chest wall is mainly soft cartilage, accounting for the sternal indrawing seen in conditions like RDS.
Auscultation: bronchial breath sounds are normal but fine crackles (crepitations) after the first few hours of life are not

(ii) Pulse rate, volume, and presence of femoral pulses to exclude coarctation; detection of full peripheral pulses, e.g. dorsalis pedis in patent ductus arteriosus

(iii) Heart examination (p. 92). Ensure silence during auscultation, using nipple or teat if necessary

6. *Abdomen*
This may be distended, and enlargement of liver (normally 2–3 cm below the right costal margin) or asymmetry due to tumours often easily seen. Gently palpate in a stroking motion from below upwards to detect them.

The kidneys can best be felt by a gentle pincer action (like squeezing a squash ball) between the thumb anteriorly and the fingers behind, supporting the back.

Listen for bowel sounds

7. *Genitals*
Always check for ambiguity (p. 39).

In boys born at term the scrotum is large and hydrocoeles that resolve by a year are common.

In girls a creamy white discharge from the vagina often becomes bloody after the first 2 days and resolves in 2–3 days due to oestrogen withdrawal; vaginal skin tags are common

8. *Anus*
Check patency and reflex tone

9. *Lower limbs*
Postural talipes is normal, but a foot that cannot move into the correct position on tickling, or spontaneously, and cannot be overcorrected by passive manipulation, requires an orthopaedic opinion.

Check the number of digits

10. *Back*
Mongolian blue spot is normal; look for spinal deformity, spina bifida or overlying naevus/hairy patch; sacral dimple is common and is rarely a sinus, and therefore needs no action

11. *Neurology*
Eyes are examined, made easier by sitting the baby up. A unilateral small pupil with ptosis (Horner's syndrome) may occur with upper limb weakness (Klumpke's palsy) from damage to cervical nerves C7,8,T1

Neurological findings are influenced by alertness, satiety (hours before/after feed) and intercurrent illness
(*i*) *Behaviour*:

a. apathy	drugs, asphyxia, sepsis, metabolic upset
b. irritability	hungry, drug withdrawal,
c. jittery	asphyxia/birth injury, sepsis, hypoglycaemia, hypocalcaemia

(*ii*) *Movement*:
   a. asymmetry, with lack of movement of one side of the body in hemisyndromes due to asphxia/birth injury
   b. floppy frog posture (p. 12) in prematurity, acute illness, cerebral injury from asphyxia/birth injury
   c. hypertonic, extended arched body with fisting, in cerebral injury, drug withdrawal, fits, kernicterus

(*iii*) *Cranial nerves*:

II	Turns to diffuse light, blinks at bright light. Opticokinetic nystagmus is elicited by holding the baby on his back on your outstretched arms, hands supporting the occiput, and you gently turning slowly clockwise.
Vestibular VIII Sternomastoid XI	The baby's head rotates towards the direction of travel. Both eyes
III,IV VI	deviate in that same direction (medial and lateral rectus of each eye).
II	The eyes have a slow, sweeping, following movement and a quick return phase, like that of adults, and this is generally considered to confirm cortical vision.
Vestibular VIII Other Stenormastoid XI Other IV,VI	A post-rotatory nystagmus and rotation of the head in the opposite direction occur on your spin stopping. Repeat, in the opposite, anti-clockwise direction to check eye movements.
III,IV,VI (alternative method)	Doll's eye response is the turning of the eyes in the opposite direction to that which the head is turned during examination. Persistent squint is abnormal, but transient squint when drowsy is not.
III	Look for ptosis, and pupillary constriction to light.
V	Rooting reflex is obtained by touching each cheek. The head turns to the side stimulated.
VII	Grimace or crying. The corner of the mouth is pulled over towards the normal side, the weak side remaining at rest.

Auditory VIII	Startle to hand clap, quieting on being talked to or to the shake of a baby rattle.
IX,X	Gag reflex present and uvula remains in midline.
XII	Vigorous sucking/stripping action by the tongue

(*iv*) *Primitive reflexes*
  a. The Moro reflex: weakness or absence of abduction and return to flexion is a useful sign in:
    one arm e.g. Erb's palsy of cervical nerves 5,6,
    both arms e.g. bilateral Erb's.
    Arm and leg same side in hemiplegia
    Note the Moro may disappear in cerebral injury
  b. Asymmetric tonic neck reflex (ATNR) should not be obligatory i.e. if baby gets 'stuck' in the ATNR this is abnormal and due to raised intracranial pressure, asphyxia or cerebral palsy
  c. Walking reflex may be impaired by sciatic nerve or spinal cord damage. Tendon reflexes are normally brisk and symmetrical

(*v*) *Tone and power* (Term infant)
  a. Pull to sit using the palmar grasp. The arms, trunk and head flex forward. Lack of flexion or marked head 'lag' is abnormal, except in an angry baby!
  b. Sitting up, the chin should rise off the chest and not snap backwards in uncontrolled extension
  c. Pick up the baby, lying prone, your hand under the abdomen. The head and back should be in line horizontally, hips and knees gently flexed

Causes of hypotonia and weakness include:
1. Prematurity
2. Drugs given mother (remember breast milk) or baby
3. Acute illness e.g. sepsis, shock, cardiorespiratory stress, intraventricular haemorrhage
4. Asphyxia
5. Neurological conditions, e.g. postictal state, meningitis, Prader-Willi syndrome, dystrophia myotonica

(*vi*) *Gestational age assessment*
  Based on the identification of certain physical characteristics, neurological or reflex responses present after different periods of gestation. Commonly used are:
  a. Appearance of certain reflexs (Robinson 1966) by weeks of gestation

Reflex	Absence	Presence
Pupils constrict to light	<31	28+
Awake infant's head turns to light	?	32+
Blink on tapping root of nose (Glabella tap)	<34	32+
Flexion of arms or neck on pulling to sit	<36	33+
Trunk follows turning of head	<37	34+

   b. Rapid physical assessment (Parkin et al 1976)
      A score based on 4 most reliable physical characteristics:
         skin colour
         ear firmness
         breast size
         skin texture
      Accuracy: to within 18 days in 95%
   c. Combined neurological and physical scoring system of
      Dubowitz et al (1970)
      Accuracy: to within 14 days in 95%
  Sources of error in the use of a, b and c
  Neurological: any condition or drug likely to depress or
    excite infant's brain: applies to methods a and c
  Physical: SFD and LFD may have inappropriately 'mature'
    features e.g. dry flaky skin, many plantar creases;
    and 'immature' ones, e.g. lark of ear cartilage,
    subcutaneous fat, breast tissue and growth of external
    genitalia: applies to b and c

12. Hip examination (Fig. 1)
   (i) Place the infant on a firm, flat surface, on his/her back.
      Ensure he/she is relaxed. Adduct and flex the hips and
      knees, then abduct them fully, looking for:
      (a) limitation of abduction in either hip (Fig. 1a)
      (b) a 'jerk' interrupting the smooth arc (Fig. 1bi)
      (c) a 'clunk' as the head relocates
  (ii) 'Telescope' the flexed thigh, abducted 45 degrees, in
      towards the acetabulum, the pelvis held firmly with the
      other hand (Fig. 1bii). Examine each hip separately
  (iii) Finally, again adduct the flexed hips and knees, and
      internally rotate the hips so that the dorsum of each foot
      faces the other. Thumbs on inner thighs, index and middle
      fingers on outer (lesser and greater trochanters
      respectively), press vertically downwards to dislocate the
      hips (Fig. 1c). Now abduct and externally rotate the thighs
      so the soles now face each other, meanwhile pressing
      upwards with the fingers. As the hip returns a 'clunk' is felt
      (Fig. 1d).
        Clicks arise from ligaments moving at hip and knee and
      are not generally thought significant

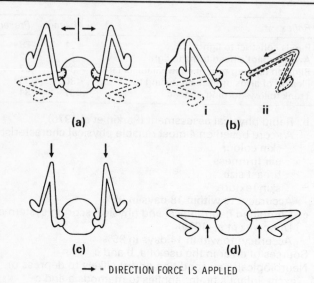

Fig. 1

→ = DIRECTION FORCE IS APPLIED

REFERENCES

Dubowitz L, Dubowitz V, Goldberg C 1970 Clinical assessment of gestational age in the newborn infant. Journal of Pediatrics 77: 1–10

Parkin J M, Hey E N, Clowes J S 1976 Rapid assessment of gestational age at birth. Archives of Disease in Childhood 51: 259–263

Robinson R J 1966 Assessment of gestational age by neurological examination. Archives of Disease in Childhood 41: 437–447

PROBLEMS OF THE LOW BIRTHWEIGHT INFANT

Of the 7% of all babies born weighing less than 2.5 kg, 60% are premature and 40% are small for dates. Further categorisation is by weight into the very low birthweight baby (VLBW) below 1500 g and the extremely low birthweight baby (ELBW) of less than 1000 g, for the purpose of identifying and documenting the high risk/dependency/cost/morbidity and mortality groups.

PREMATURITY

Born before 37 weeks' gestation

Causes
1. Unknown
2. Uterus
    (i) Abnormal e.g. cervical incompetence, double uterus
    (ii) Uterine distension e.g. twins, polyhydramnios
    (iii) Premature rupture of membranes, includes (i)
3. Maternal
    (i) School age
    (ii) Previous premature delivery
    (iii) Closely spaced pregnancies
    (iv) Acute maternal illness, drug addiction
4. Fetal: congenital malformation, infection
5. Environmental: poverty
6. Therapeutic: rhesus isoimmunisation, diabetes, fetal distress
   fetoscopy(?)

PROBLEMS OF THE PREMATURE

Early
1. Immaturity
    (i) Respiration
        a. Central control unstable (apnoea)
        b. Surfactant deficiency (respiratory distress syndrome)
        c. Alveolar–arteriolar gradient in the ELBW due to
           columnar epithelium, vascular beds underdeveloped
    (ii) Cardiovascular: bradycardias, hypotension, cardiac failure
         from patent ductus arteriosus from early fluid excess or
         reopens with hypoxia, anaemia
    (iii) Feeding: absent gag reflex before 34 weeks, functional ileus
    (iv) Liver: jaundice
2. Hypothermia: lack of brown fat and subcutaneous fat layer
3. Hypoglycaemia: lack of liver glycogen stores
4. Intraventricular haemorrhage: the less mature the more likely
5. Infection
6. Necrotising enterocolitis
7. Iatrogenic (see p. 27)
8. Hyponatraemia: 'salt wasting' kidneys of the VLBW

Later
1. Bonding failure
2. Anaemia
    a. Early dilutional = normochromic at 4–6 weeks
    b. Late nutritional = hypochromic at 8–12 weeks
    c. Haemolytic = folic acid deficient, vitamin E deficiency
3. 'Rickets of prematurity': probably inadequate phosphorous
   and/or calcium intake in very low birthweight infants. Classical
   rickets due to lack of vitamin D more likely in premature infants
   because of rapid growth rate

4. Persistent patent ductus arteriosus: early fluid overload
5. Oxygen toxicity: retrolental fibroplasia, bronchopulmonary dysplasia (mechanical ventilation also implicated)
6. Brain damage: cerebral palsy, hydrocephalus from intraventricular haemorrhage
7. Growth potential: may be diminished in the ELBW

SMALL FOR DATES (SFD/LFD)

Definition
Below the 10th centile for weight. These infants may be symmetrically small in all body proportions or light for dates, i.e. length and head circumference above the 10th centile.

Causes
1. Symmetrically small: early interference with fetal growth before 25 weeks' gestation
   (i) Fetal
      a. Chromosomal abnormalities e.g. trisomy 21, 13–15, 18, XO
      b. Congenital abnormality
      c. Fetal infection: cytomegalovirus, toxoplasmosis, rubella, herpes simplex, malaria, syphilis
   (ii) Maternal
      Drugs e.g. chronic alcoholism, heroin addiction
2. Small in height and/or weight, usually with sparing of head growth. Attributed to onset of chronic intrauterine malnutrition after 24 weeks' gestation
   (i) Maternal
      a. Malnutrition, race, social disadvantage etc
      b. Hypoxaemia e.g. smoking, high altitude, cyanotic cardiorespiratory disease
   (ii) Placental insufficiency
      a. Maternal vascular disease e.g. renal, essential hypertension, collagen disease, sickle cell, toxaemia
      b. Abnormal placentation with reduced placental weight and cellularity
      c. Placental infarction
   (iii) Inadequate space e.g. multiple pregnancy, bicornuate uterus

PROBLEMS OF THE SMALL FOR DATES INFANT

1. Hypoxia
   (i) Intrauterine death during pregnancy or labour
   (ii) Polycythaemia
   (iii) Meconium aspiration causing pneumonia

2. Hypoglycaemia: inadequate glycogen stores, jittery, increased hunger drive
3. Hypothermia: lack of subcutaneous fat
4. Polycythaemia: results in jaundice, thromboses in the brain, heart failure, pulmonary haemorrhage
5. Congenital/chromosomal/infection problems: i.e. *examine very carefully*!

PROBLEMS OF THE LFD INFANT

1. Intrauterine: chronic hypoxia, intrauterine death
2. Intrapartum
    (i) Acute or chronic hypoxia → death
    (ii) Meconium aspiration
3. Postpartum
    (i) Hypoglycaemia in first 12 hours
    (ii) Temperature instability, increased calorie requirements
    (iii) Polycythaemia: jaundice, thromboses, cardiac failure
    (iv) Pulmonary haemorrhage
    (v) Behavioural jitteriness, excessive/diminished feeding ability

CONDITIONS ASSOCIATED WITH HYDRAMNIOS

1. Intrauterine death
2. Anencephaly
3. High intestinal obstruction
4. Cord tight round neck
5. Down's syndrome

CONDITIONS ASSOCIATED WITH OLIGOHYDRAMNIOS

1. Kidney agenesis, dysplasia, infantile polycystic kidney
2. Renal tract outlet obstruction, e.g. posterior urethral valves
3. Chronic amniotic fluid leak
4. Intrauterine growth retardation
5. Post-term

CONDITIONS ASSOCIATED WITH THE ONSET OF RESPIRATORY DISTRESS SYNDROME (RDS)

1. Prematurity
2. Asphyxia, intrapartum aspiration
3. Second twin
4. Severe rhesus isoimmunisation
5. Maternal factors
    (i) Antepartum or intrapartum haemorrhage
    (ii) Caesarean delivery without labour
    (iii) Diabetes mellitus
6. Previous sibling with RDS

BIRTH TRAUMA

1. *Swellings and the usual time of identification:*
    (i) Caput: at birth
    (ii) Cephalhaematoma: 2–4 days old
    (iii) Fractured clavicle: 1–20 + days
    (iv) Sternomastoid tumour: 7–20 + days. Intrauterine posture also a cause
    (v) Fat necrosis: 3–14 days
2. *Common nerve palsies, usually identified at birth*
    (i) Facial nerve, peripheral: asymmetrical crying face, open eye. (Absence of depressor anguli oris is associated with congenital heart disease, i.e. think of it if only mouth affected)
    (ii) Erb's palsy C5,6. Waiter's tip posture
    (iii) Klumpke's palsy C7,8,T1. Claw hand, flexed elbow (plus Horner's syndrome if stellate ganglion involved)
    (iv) Spinal cord transection between C2–8, often bilateral, with Erb's palsy, respiratory distress, and isolated cord with spasticity and anaesthesia below the level of the lesion
    (v) Sciatic nerve, S1–4, adopts foot drop ± sensory loss on dorsum of the foot

CAUSES OF FAILURE TO ESTABLISH RESPIRATION

1. Neurological
    (i) Maternal medication/sedation
    (ii) Asphyxia/birth injury
    (iii) Prematurity
2. Respiratory
    (i) Laryngeal spasm due to vigorous pharyngeal suction, laryngeal atresia/obstruction
    (ii) Pneumothorax
    (iii) Massive meconium aspiration
    (iv) Small lungs, e.g. Potter's syndrome of absent kidney function, oligohydramnios, pulmonary hypoplasia and 'squashed baby'
    (v) Diaphragmatic hernia
3. Circulatory = shock from blood loss
    (i) Internal: ruptured organ, into muscles, subaponeurotic
    (ii) Maternal
    (iii) Twin to twin
4. Metabolic
    (i) Hypoglycaemia
    (ii) Acidosis

HYPEROXIA TEST

Abolition of cyanosis, present while breathing room air, by breathing 100% oxygen makes parenchymal lung disease likely and congenital heart disease or large vascular shunts unlikely

CAUSES OF RESPIRATORY DISTRESS, APNOEA AND CYANOSIS

1. Respiratory
   (i) Parenchymal: respiratory distress syndrome (RDS), meconium aspiration, pneumonia, pneumothorax
   (ii) Congenital structural, upper airway: hypoplastic jaw + cleft palate (Pierre Robin's syndrome), choanal atresia, oesophageal atresia
   (iii) Congenital structural, lower airway: lung hypoplasia, lobar emphysema, cysts, diaphragmatic hernia
2. Cardiac
   (i) Cardiac failure
   (ii) Congenital heart disease
   (iii) Persistent fetal ciculation: full term, moderately asphyxiated baby, normal heart and lungs, raised pulmonary vascular resistance
3. Neurological
   (i) Asphyxia/birth injury; CVA (intraventricular haemorrhage); drugs
   (ii) Epilepsy i.e. seizures
   (iii) Floppy i.e. primary muscle disease e.g. dystrophia myotonica
4. Metabolic: hypoglycaemia, acidosis
5. Polycythaemia, anaemia (acyanotic)
6. Methaemoglobinaemia

CAUSES OF APATHY, APNOEA, IRRITABILITY, SEIZURE

1. Drugs and drug withdrawal
2. Asphyxia/birth injury
   Immature respiratory centre in premature infants
3. Infection, congenital and acquired
4. Metabolic: low glucose, sodium, calcium, magnesium, acidosis, kernicterus, inborn errors (e.g. maple syrup urine disease, galactosaemia, degenerative disease, lactic acidosis) pyridoxine deficiency and dependency syndromes
5. Intraventricular haemorrhage: premature, vitamin K deficiency, thrombocytopenia (p. 23), atrioventricular malformation
6. Fifth day fits
7. Congenital brain malformation, chromosome abnormality, neoplasm
8. Familial: neurodermatoses (tuberous sclerosis, incontinentia pigmentii), familial neonatal convulsions

(*Aid to memory*: **A**sphyxia, **B**irth injury, **C**ongenital/chromosomal, **D**rugs, **E**pilepsy (familial neonatal fits), **F**ifth day fits, **G**lucose and other metabolic causes, **H**aemorrhage, **I**mmaturity, **I**nfection)
Current interest surrounds apnoea without obvious cause, usually in the second week, and possible 'cot death'. Provisionally divided into:

1. Central, or with open airway: O_2 and CO_2 responsiveness reduced, ↑ temp, reflux, ↑ laryngeal reflex to water/cow's milk etc
2. Obstructive, or with closed airway: Pierre Robin's syndrome, neck posture, hypopharyngeal/laryngeal closure, reflux
3. Mixed: both patterns are seen

HAZARDS OF CONTINUOUS DISTENDING PRESSURE (CPAP), (PEEP) ETC

Pneumothorax
Interstitial emphysema
Intracranial haemorrhage
Hypotension
Barotrauma to lungs

CAUSES OF BRONCHOPULMONARY DYSPLASIA

1. Extreme prematurity
2. Oxygen therapy
3. Barotrauma (damage due to ventilator pressures)
4. Fluid overload and patent ductus arteriosus
5. Infection/retained secretions

CONDITIONS ASSOCIATED WITH PULMONARY HAEMORRHAGE

1. Light or small for dates
2. Rhesus isoimmunisation
3. Infant of diabetic mother
4. Pneumonia
5. Asphyxia
6. Cerebral oedema
7. Acute left ventricular failure
8. Drugs: tolazoline

CAUSES OF JAUNDICE

Clinically recognised at 100 μmol/1
'Direct' or conjugated bilirubin should be less than 25 μmol/1
* = conditions in which 'direct' bilirubin is raised

1. First day
   (i) Rhesus isoimmunisation, occasionally ABO incompatability
   (ii) Infection*, congenital (TORCH) and acquired
2. First week
   (i) Physiological
   (ii) Haemolytic
       a. blood group incompatibility (* after exchange transfusions)
       b. red cell abnormality, e.g. hereditary spherocytosis
       c. enzyme deficiency: glucose-6-phosphate dehydrogenase deficiency, pyruvate kinase, glutathione synthetase deficiency
       d. Vitamin K excess, or water soluble vitamin K
   (iii) Polycythaemia: small for dates, late clamping of cord, fetomaternal and fetal–fetal transfusion
   (iv) Extravisated blood reabsorption from bruises, cephalhaematoma, swallowed maternal blood
   (v) Infection*, congenital and acquired
   (vi) Gut obstruction: ileus, Hirschsprung's disease
   (vii) Metabolic
       a. minor contributory: oxytocics, hypoglycaemia, dehydration
       b. moderate and rare: Lucey-Driscoll syndrome
       c. major but rare: Crigler-Najjar (Arias type 1) and type 2, both glucuronyl transferase deficiency
3. Late onset after 1 week
   (i) Breast milk jaundice
   (ii) Infection*: urinary tract infection, herpes, hepatitis
   (iii) Metabolic
       a. parenteral alimentation in the VLBW*
       b. hypothyroidism
       c. Gilbert's familial non-haemolytic jaundice
       d. Cystic fibrosis
       e. Alpha-1-antitrypsin deficiency*
       f. Galactosaemia*
   (iv) Biliary atresia*/neonatal hepatitis syndrome*

Alternative strategy
1. Pre-hepatic: haemolytic, extravisated blood, infection
2. Hepatic: physiological, congenital infection, hypothyroidism, neonatal hepatitis syndrome
3. Post-hepatic: biliary atresia

ANAEMIA

At birth a healthy mature infant's venous haemoglobin (Hb) is 19 g/dl; a premature infant's Hb is 16 g/dl
Anaemia: less than 14 g/dl in the first week

Causes
1. Haemorrhage
   (i) Into mother/twin
   (ii) Into baby: trauma, vitamin K deficiency, anticoagulants to mother
   (iii) Revealed: cord and placenta accidents, circumcision
2. Haemolysis
   (i) Infection, profound acidosis
   (ii) Rhesus (direct Coombs' test positive), ABO etc
   (iii) Red cell defects: G-6-PD, spherocytosis (p. 127)
   (iv) Haemoglobinopathies: Hb Barts, etc
   (v) Drugs: vitamin K, aniline dye
3. Iatrogenic (blood taking)
4. Inadequate production (rare), due to hypoplastic RBC anaemia (Blackfan-Diamond), or replaced by congenital tumour (neuroblastoma), leukaemia or histiocytosis (Letterer-Siwe)

CAUSES OF HAEMOLYTIC DISEASE

1. Direct Coombs' test strongly positive
   (i) Rh D negative mother, Rh D positive fetus
   (ii) Rh D positive mother, Rh c, E, e, C and Kell, Duffy, Kidd positive fetus
2. Direct Coombs' test negative or weakly positive A, B, AB in fetus of mother group O or rarely A_2
3. Direct Coombs' test negative
   (i) Infection: bacterial, congenital, viral and parasite
   (ii) RBC enzyme defects: G-6-PD, pyruvate kinase, hexokinase, galactosaemia
   (iii) Abnormal RBC morphology: congenital spherocytosis, elliptocytosis, haemoglobin Barts (stillborn)
   (iv) Congenital erythropoietic porphyria

CAUSES OF THROMBOCYTOPENIA

1. Neonatal disease
   (i) Infection: septicaemia, congenital infection, e.g. rubella, cytomegalovirus, herpes simplex, toxoplasmosis
   (ii) Consumption: asphyxia, placental abruption, trauma, acidosis, respiratory distress syndrome
   (iii) Severe rhesus isoimmunisation
   (iv) Maternal
      a. Platelet antibodies: ITP, SLE, isoimmunisation
      b. Drugs e.g. thiazides
   (v) Rare: hyperglycinaemia, leukaemia
2. Dilution: exchange transfusion
3. Loss: haemorrhage

CAUSES OF HYPOGLYCAEMIA

See p. 6 for normal values
1. Delayed or inadequate feeds
2. Inadequate stores
    (i) Prematurity
    (ii) Small for dates
    (iii) Inborn errors of carbohydrate metabolism e.g.
        galactosaemia, fructose intolerance
3. Increased requirement
    (i) Stress: infection, RDS, hypothermia
    (ii) Hyperinsulinism: infant of a diabetic mother,
        erythroblastosis, nesidioblastosis, Beckwith's syndrome
    (iii) Drugs: maternal tolbutamide etc
    (iv) Idiopathic

CAUSES OF HYPOCALCAEMIA

(Less than 1.8 mmol/l)
1. Early, 0–3 days: low calcium, normal phosphate
    (i) Prematures
    (ii) Asphyxia
    (iii) Small for dates
    (iv) Stress e.g. RDS, sepsis, surgical
    (v) Infant of diabetic mother
    (vi) Alkali infusion, exchange transfusion
2. Late, 4–21 days: low calcium and/or magnesium, elevated
    phosphate
    (i) Cow's milk
    (ii) Maternal hyperparathyroidism, vitamin D deficiency,
        osteoporosis, renal disease
    (iii) Di George's syndrome (p. 133)

CAUSES OF VOMITING

1. First 1–3 days
    (i) Feeding problem
    (ii) Gastric irritation, swallowed blood
    (iii) Obstruction: duodenal atresia (double bubble on X-ray),
        stricture or web, annular pancreas, Ladd's bands, mid-gut
        rotation, meconium ileus, meconium plug, Hirschsprung's
        disease, anal atresia
    (iv) Functional ileus in premature, stressed
    (v) Infection
    (vi) Neurological: asphyxia/birth injury, intraventricular
        haemorrhage

2. *End of first week*
   (i) Hiatus hernia
   (iii) Infection
   (iii) Necrotising enterocolitis
   (iv) Metabolic: renal failure, inborn errors of metabolism, e.g. congenital adrenal hyperplasia (p. 50), galactosaemia, organic acidaemias, lactic acidosis
   (v) Obstructive: pyloric stenosis, volvulus, anal stenosis, small left colon, Hirschsprung's disease

CAUSES OF ACUTE ABDOMINAL DISTENSION

1. Air swallowing: feeding, tracheo-oesophageal fistula
2. Intestinal
   (i) 'Functional ileus': premature, asphyxia, stress
   (ii) Obstruction: pylorus, duodenum, volvulus
   (iii) Necrotising enterocolitis
   (iv) Meconium ileus
   (v) Hirschsprung's disease
3. Congestive cardiac failure
4. Tension pneumothorax

CAUSES OF DELAY IN PASSING MECONIUM

1. On the first day:
   (i) Organic obstruction: anal stenosis or atresia, vesicorectal malformations, extrinsic rectal pressure, neonatal small left colon
   (ii) Motility disorders: prematurity, opiates, Hirschsprung's disease
   (iii) Metabolic: hypothermia, cystic fibrosis
   (iv) Meconium plug
2. Delay in passing stool on subsequent days also include:
   (i) Underfeeding, vomiting
   (ii) Breast feeding, simple constipation
   (iii) Hypothyroidism

CAUSES OF HAEMATEMESIS

1. Swallowed maternal blood
2. Gastritis
3. Oesophagitis
4. Peptic 'stress' ulceration, duplication, Meckel's diverticulum
5. Iatrogenic trauma — e.g. nasogastric tubes, airways
6. Coagulation defect: vitamin K deficiency, consumption of factors, low platelet count
7. Necrotising enterocolitis

8. Vascular abnormality: haemangioma, areteriovenous malformation, telangiectasia
9. Volvulus — bleeding from damaged bowel

CAUSES OF BLOOD IN THE STOOL

1. Swallowed maternal blood
2. Infection
3. Necrotising enterocolitis
4. Trauma, local e.g. hard stool, thermometer
5. Cow's milk allergy
6. Haemorrhagic disease of the newborn (vitamin K deficiency)
7. Acid ulceration: stress, hiatus hernia, Meckel's diverticulum
8. No cause found

CAUSES OF ABDOMINAL SWELLING

1. Renal: hydronephrosis or multicystic kidney together cause 80%; posterior urethral valves, polycystic kidney, renal vein thrombosis, pelvic kidney, tumour e.g. Wilms'
2. Hepatic: cardiac failure, subcapsular haematoma, haemangiomas, lymphangiomas, supradiaphragmatic pressure e.g. tension pneumothorax, cysts, small thorax
3. Spleen: infection, rhesus isoimmunisation, subcapsular haematoma, hepatic causes
4. Intestinal: meconium ileus, meconium pseudocysts, duplications, volvulus, intussusception, Hirschsprung's disease
5. Adrenal: haemorrhage, neuroblastoma (commonest congenital tumour)
6. Ovarian cysts, hydrocolpos
7. Teratoma

CAUSES OF ACUTE RENAL FAILURE

1. Congenital (80%)
   (i) Agenesis, dysplasia of kidneys
   (ii) Obstruction
   (iii) Nephrotic syndrome
2. Hypotension: usually blood loss, asphyxia, coarctation of aorta
3. Urinary tract infection, septicaemia
4. Haemolytic uraemic syndrome
5. Renal vein thrombosis, renal artery thrombosis

CAUSES OF CARDIAC FAILURE — see page 101

GUTHRIE TEST ROUTINELY PERFORMED BETWEEN 6TH AND 14TH DAY OF LIFE

Screens for:
  Phenylketonuria
  Hypermethioninaemia
  Histidinaemia
Some laboratories also look for:
  TSH level
  Hyperleucinaemia (in maple syrup urine disease)
  Galactosaemia
  Tyrosinaemia
  Glucose-6-phosphate dehydrogenese deficiency

Errors
1. If infant is receiving antibiotics directly or via mother's breast milk (kills Bacillus subtilis, the test organism)
2. Not receiving adequate milk feeds
3. Hypothyroidism is due to hypopituitarism in 1 in 10 hypothyroid babies and will remain undetected as TSH not elevated

CAUSES OF SEIZURES (see p. 65 for relationship by age at onset)

1. Traumatic: birth injury, asphyxia
2. Metabolic
     (i) Hypoglycaemia
     (ii) Low Ca^{++}, Mg^{++}
     (iii) Water intoxication, low Na^+
     (iv) Elevated bilirubin (kernicterus), Na^+
     (vi) Pyridoxine dependency or deficiency
3. Drug
     (i) Withdrawal
     (ii) Intoxication, e.g. local anaesthetic
4. Infection: congenital and acquired
5. Intracranial haemorrhage
     (i) Prematurity
     (ii) Haematological: vitamin K, ↓ platelets, DIC
     (iii) Cerebral arterio-venous malformations
6. Genetic
     (i) Metabolic errors, e.g. maple syrup urine disease, galactosaemia, lactic acidosis, degenerative diseases
     (ii) Neurodermatoses: tuberous sclerosis, incontinentia pigmentii
     (iii) Familial neonatal convulsion
7. Congenital cerebral malformations, neoplasm

CAUSES OF IATROGENIC DISEASE

Historical
1. Delayed feeding of prematures: *early* hypoglycaemia, *later* increased incidence of cerebral palsy
2. Deliberate hypothermia, incorrectly thought to reduce oxygen requirements. Increased mortality
3. Jaundice
   (i) Water soluble vitamin K causing haemolysis
   (ii) Drugs displacing bilirubin from albumin causing kernicterus, e.g. sulphonamides
   (iii) Drug inhibition of glucuronidation by novobiocin

Still topical
1. Retrolental fibroplasia: oxygen toxicity plays a part
2. Chloramphenicol excess: 'grey baby syndrome' — shock due to cardiovascular collapse, fits
3. Excessive separation of parents and infant

FURTHER READING

Cloherty J P, Stark A R 1986 (eds) Manual of neonatal care. Little, Brown, Boston

The Newborn. I, II 1986 Pediatric Clinics of North America 33(2, 3). Saunders, Philadelphia

Roberton N R C and Grundy G M 1986 Lecture notes on neonatology. Blackwell, Oxford

Screening for the detection of congenital dislocation of the hip. A special report 1986 Archives of Diseases in Childhood 61: 921–926

Growth and nutritional requirements

NORMAL GROWTH: SOME CLINICAL RULES OF THUMB

1. Fetal weight: 1.1 kg at 28 weeks, 2.2 kg at 34 weeks, 3.3 kg at 40 weeks
2. Infant weight gain: 30 g/day (1 oz) from the 10th day
   Birth weight × 2 by 5 months
   Birth weight × 3 by one year
3. Childhood expected weight
   Weight in kg = 3 × age in years + 4
4. Milestones in height
   Birth   50 cm
   One year   75 cm
   4 years   100 cm
   Middle childhood: 5–7.5 cm per year
5. Occipitofrontal circumference
   Birth   35 cm
   One year   47 cm (i.e. +12 months)
   Two years   49 cm (i.e. +2 years)
6. Tooth eruption, onset to completion
   Primary dentition   6 months to 2 years
   Permanent dentition   6 years to 12 years
   Third molars   20 years +

NUTRITIONAL REQUIREMENTS FOR MAINTENANCE AND GROWTH

1. *Water*. Determined by
   (i) A relatively high body water content: 80% at birth, 65% by 6 months, 60% in the adult
   (ii) Renal concentrating ability is age related (p.140) and less in infancy
   (iii) Insensible water loss is high: large surface area relative to mass in infancy

Neonate	150 ml/kg/day	After 1 week of age until weaning begins at 4 months post-term orally as milk
Premature up to	200 ml/kg/day	
< 10 kg	100 ml/kg/day	Oral or intravenous as water
10–20 kg	50 ml/kg/day	
> 20 kg	20 ml/kg/day	

2. *Calories*
   (i) Up to one year: 460 kJ (110 kcal) per day for each kg body weight. Prematures up to 580 kJ (140 kcal) per day
   (ii) Subsequent years: 4200 kJ (1000 kcal) + 420 kJ (100 kcal) for each year of life
   (iii) Calculate according to *expected* weight for *gestational* age and each year of life. Remember that 150 ml of milk contains 460 kJ (110 kcal)
   (iv) Weaning: first solids introduced from 3–6 months, unmodified cow's milk from 6 months
3. *Minerals*
   Sodium, potassium, chloride   2 mmol/kg/day
   Calcium, phosphate   5 mmol/kg/day
   Elemental iron   1–2 mg/kg/day
4. *Protein*
   Term infants   2 g/kg/day
   Prematures   2–4 g/kg/day
5. *Vitamins*. Recommended daily intake in the first year
   Term   A 1500 IU
                       C   30 mg
                       D   400 IU
   Premature (very low birth-weight)
                       A, B, C as above
                       D 800 IU
                       E 15 mg   } for 2–6 months
                       Folic acid 50 μ
6. *Fluoride*. Daily supplement given is related to tap water content and infant's age. (Optimal fluoride concentration is one part per million (ppm) in tap water.) Most toothpastes now contain fluoride

HAZARDS OF COW'S MILK FEEDING

1. Psychological, e.g. less satisfying, disappointed if unable to breast feed
2. Infection
   (i) Preparation
   (ii) Lack of anti-infective factors
3. Electrocyte disorders: hypocalcaemia, hyponatraemia
4. Allergy: eczema, asthma, migraine, urticaria, anaphylaxis
5. Obesity

6. Cow's milk protein intolerance: infantile colic, coeliac like, acute colitis
7. Anaemia: occult bleeding
8. Intestinal obstruction from curds
9. Controversial: cot death, ulcerative colitis, multiple sclerosis, coronary artery disease

ADDITIONAL HAZARDS OF FORMULA MILKS

1. Preparation
   (i) Overconcentration: hypernatraemia (historical?), obesity
   (ii) Overdilution: marasmus
   (iii) Anaemia, as symptom of cow's milk protein allergy
2. Deficiencies
   (i) Pyridoxine: convulsions (historical)
   (ii) Linoleic acid: rash (historical)
   (iii) Vitamin E: haemolytic anaemia

ADVERSE FACTORS IN BREAST FEEDING

1. Underfeeding
2. Deficiencies: vitamin D, vitamin K
3. Hypoproteinaemia and hyponatraemia in premature infants
4. Drugs excreted: sedatives, tranquilliser, etc
5. Drugs to be avoided completely: antithyroid, antimitotic, chloramphenicol, ergot, meprobamate, aspirin in high dosage, iodides, unmonitored lithium

FURTHER READING

Wood C, Walker Smith J 1982 MacKeith's infant feeding and feeding difficulties. 6th edn. Churchill Livingstone, Edinburgh

GROWTH

Growth curves are derived from longitudinal data (repeated measurements at intervals), and cross-sectional data (a single measurement of many individuals of different ages). Longitudinal reflect individual patterns, cross-sectional smooth out individual variation. The curves are divided by centiles, e.g. 97th centile 97% of population are smaller, 3% are larger at that age

Measurement
Single measurements of height and weight allow a static comparison with the rest of the population using a standard growth chart.

Repeated measurements allow assessment of the rate of growth or growth velocity. The minimum interval between such measurements is 3 months using an accurate stadiometer, by the same experienced observer

Use of charts (Figs 2–5)
1. Distance chart: growth in height or weight achieved year on year. A single measurement allows a static comparison
2. Growth velocity chart: growth rate in centimetres per year, requires at least two measurements three or more months apart. For example, a child whose height is on the 3rd centile year on year has a growth velocity close to the 50th centile. A child of average height with growth velocity on the 3rd centile will quickly show a fall off in growth

Parental height comparison
This will show whether the child is on the expected mid-parental centile
1. Roughly calculated from the standard chart as follows:
   Boys (i) plot mother's height on the right hand margin
         (ii) add 12.5 cm to this, make a mark
         (iii) plot father's height
         (iv) expected height centile is midpoint between (ii) and (iii)
   Girls (i) plot father's height and deduct 12.5 cm, mark
         (ii) expected height centile is midway between the mark and mother's height
   95% confidence limit for this estimate is 8 cm either side of the midpoint
2. *Parent allowed for chart* is more accurate. The child is compared against standards for children with parents of the same height. Thus for a child on the 3rd centile, with parents also on the 3rd centile for the general population, he will be on the 50th centile on this chart

ASSESSMENT OF SKELETAL MATURITY
1. Greulich-Pyle atlas: by comparing a hand and wrist X-ray of a child with standard X-ray of ossification at different chronological ages, a 'bone age' is obtained
2. TW2 method of Tanner and Whitehouse: by giving a numerical score for amount of ossification to each bone of the hand and wrist, a composite score is obtained and plotted on a centile chart for the child's age, like height and weight. Conversion of TW2 score to bone age = age at which score is on 50th centile. It is 0.8 years behind Greulich-Pyle bone age

Variations in skeletal maturity
1. Normal bone age i.e. same as chronological age, in short stature of familial or genetic cause
2. Delay indicates extra potential for growth e.g. a 16 year old with a 7 year old's bone age has a similar, but not necessarily equal, growth potential to a younger child of that age
   (i) Delayed bone age proportional to actual height, i.e. the height plotted on the chart at that bone age is within expected centiles (Fig. 4a) in constitutional growth delay
   (ii) Delayed bone age, the actual height progressively falling away from expected velocity in failure to thrive (p. 35), hypothyroidism, growth hormone deficiency (Fig. 4b). Without treatment final adult height may be reduced.
3. Advanced bone age (Fig. 4c) in virilisation and precocious puberty (p. 42). Untreated it would result in premature epiphyseal fusion, with final adult height below expected, especially in boys

CATCH-UP GROWTH

This occurs for a finite period after suppression by subnutrition or severe illness and is an increased growth velocity towards expected stature (Figs. 4a,b; 5a)

GROWTH VELOCITY CHARTS

These provide information about the rate of change in height or weight, and most readily alert the clinician during observation of growth or in supervising treatment for growth disorders (Fig. 5a,b)

CAUSES OF SHORT STATURE — after Charles Brook

1. Normal looking
   (i) Normal growth velocity
      a. Low birthweight
      b. Short parents
      c. Constitutional growth delay
   (ii) Low growth velocity
      a. Psychosocial deprivation
      b. Generalised disease, e.g. malabsorption, metabolic and systemic disease (see below)
2. Distinguishing features
   (i) Disproportionate growth
      a. Short trunk, e.g. spondylo-epiphyseal dysplasia
      b. Short limbs, e.g. achondroplasia
   (ii) Growth disorder syndromes, e.g. Russell Silver syndrome, progeria, etc

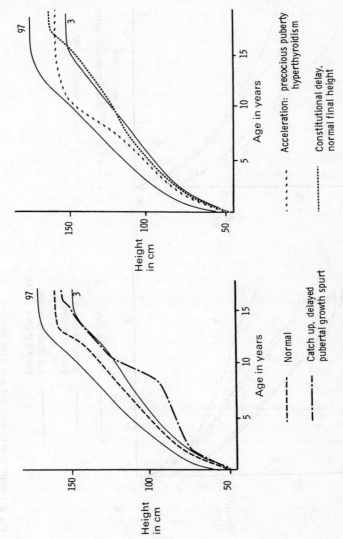

Fig. 2 Height charts with 3rd and 97th centiles

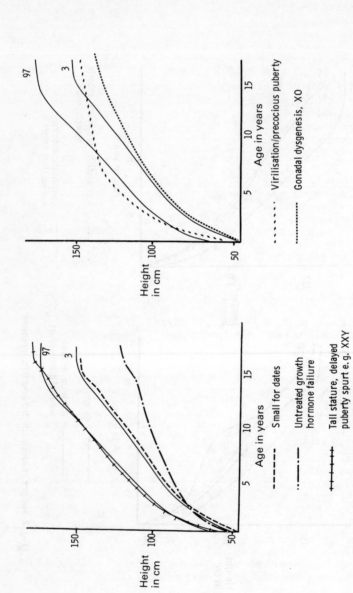

Fig. 3 Height charts with 3rd and 97th centiles

Causes of short stature — alternative strategy
1. Common causes
    (i) Undernutrition
    (ii) Constitutional: individual and familial
    (iii) Psychosocial deprivation
    (iv) Small for dates from toxaemia
    (v) Malabsorption: intestinal infection, tropical infestation, coeliac, cystic fibrosis, Hirschsprung's disease
    (vi) Mental retardation
    (vii) Iatrogenic: steroids
2. Less common causes
    (i) Systemic disease: cyanotic congenital heart disease, cystic fibrosis, severe asthma, chronic renal failure
    (ii) Chronic infection: malaria
    (iii) Skeletal disorders: achondroplasia, rickets, spinal tuberculosis
3. Rare causes
    (i) Endocrine: hypothyroidism, hypopituitarism, sexual precocity, Cushing's
    (ii) Chromosomal: XO, Down's syndrome
    (iii) Metabolic
        a. Genetic, e.g. glycogen storage
        b. Acquired, e.g. renal tubular acidosis, vitamin D induced hypercalcaemia

Causes of short sature/failure to thrive — traditional strategy
1. Subnutrition: lack/inappropriate foods, psychosocial deprivation
2. Constitutional: individual, familial
3. Low birthweight/small for dates (or as a mistake in premature infants where no allowance is made for prematurity in the first 2 years)
4. Dwarfing conditions:
    (i) Genetic e.g. achondroplasia
    (ii) Chromosomal e.g. Turner's syndrome (XO)
    (iii) Mental retardation e.g. microcephaly
    (iv) Russell–Silver syndrome
5. Systemic diseases:
    (i) Malabsorption, e.g. infective and postinfective diarrhoea (p. 116), coeliac, cystic fibrosis, Hirschsprung's disease
    (ii) Infection
    (iii) Asthma — poorly controlled/steroid excess
    (iv) Cyanotic congenital heart disease, renal failure
    (v) Endocrine e.g. hypothyroid, hypopituitary, Cushing's (including iatrogenic from steroids)

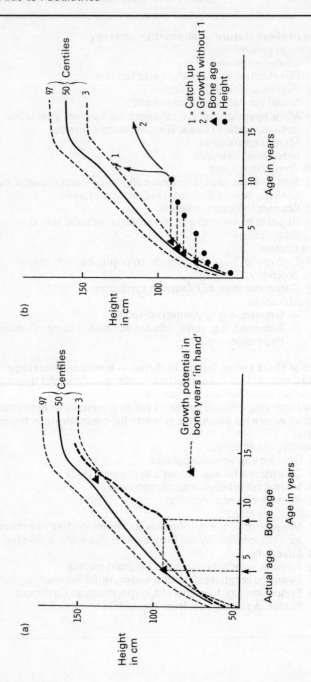

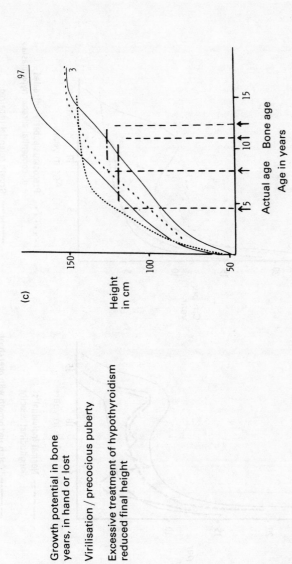

(c)

Height in cm

150

100

50

Actual age   Bone age
Age in years

5   10   15

97

3

▲——— Growth potential in bone years, in hand or lost

·········· Virilisation / precocious puberty

···· ···· Excessive treatment of hypothyroidism reduced final height

Fig. 4 Height charts using bone age

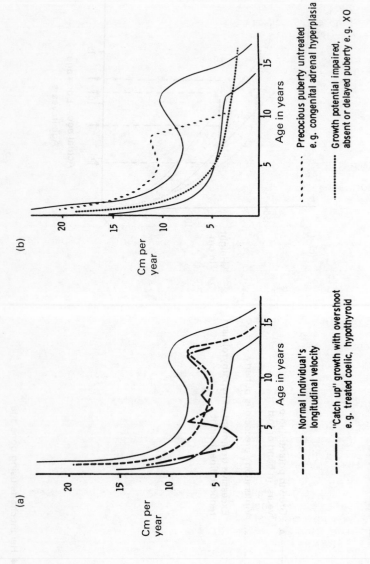

Fig. 5 Height velocity charts

CAUSES OF TALL STATURE

1. Constitutional, familial, occasionally isolated
2. *True precocious puberty (p. 42)
3. Chromosomal: XXY, XYY
4. Endocrine
   (i) Thyrotoxicosis
   (ii) Congenital adrenal hyperplasia, adrenal secreting tumours
   (iii) Gonadal secreting tumours
   (iv) Testicular feminisation
   (v) Beckwith's syndrome
5. *Hydrocephalus
6. Metabolic: Marfan's, homocystinuria
7. *Cerebral gigantism (Sotos syndrome)

AMBIGUOUS GENITALIA

Normal fetal sexual differentiation

Male: H-Y antigen on Y chromosome induces undifferentiated
         gonad to form testis, the Leydig and Sertoli cells of
         which are then stimulated by placental chorionic
         gonadotrophin to secrete testosterone and Mullerian
         inhibitory factor (MIF)
         (i) Testosterone → epididymis, vas deferens,
              5α   obliteration of lower
              reductase ↓ third of vagina
         (ii) Dihydrotestosterone → external male genitalia
         (iii) MIF → obliteration of uterus, Fallopian tubes, upper
              two-thirds of vagina
Female: development of female genitalia occurs if H-Y antigen is
         absent. No need of ovarian or adrenal androgen
         secretion

Causes of ambiguous genitalia

1. Virilisation of females
   (i) Congenital adrenal hyperplasia
   (ii) Androgen as drug ingestion or secreting tumour, in mother
        or after birth
2. Hermaphrodite
   (i) True hermaphrodite: 46 XX, 46 XY/46XX mosaic
   (ii) Mixed gonadal dysgenesis: usually 46 XY/45 XO mosaic
3. Feminisation of males
   (i) Undescended testes
       a. Normal
       b. XXY
       c. Anorchia

* Before premature closure of epiphyses

   (ii) Inadequate virilisation ± scrotal growth
      a. Errors in testosterone synthesis (p. 50)
      b. Testicular feminisation: complete end-organ androgen
         insensitivity
      c. Other androgen insensitivity syndromes, e.g. 5α
         reductase deficiency
  (iii) Inguinal masses: persistent Müllerian structures, testicular
         feminisation
  (iv) Micropenis
      a. Idiopathic
      b. Hypopituitarism: isolated growth hormone deficiency,
         Kalmann's, Prader-Willi
      c. Testicular: XXY rudimentary testes, errors in
         testosterone synthesis (p. 50)
      d. Androgen insensitivity
      e. Dysmorphic syndromes: Down's, Noonan's, Williams',
         Smith-Lemli-Opitz

Findings on examining these external genitalia
1. No gonads
    (i) Virilisation of female
   (ii) Feminisation of male (see 3 ii, iii above)
2. One gonad
    (i) Unilateral testicular descent in male
   (ii) True hermaphrodite or gonadal dysgenesis
3. Two gonads
    (i) Inadequate virilisation (see 3 ii, iii above)
   (ii) True hermaphrodite with bilateral ovotestes

FURTHER READING

Hughes I A 1984 Medical and psychological management of congenital
  adrenal hyperplasia. In: Anysley Green A (ed) Paediatric endocrinology in
  Clinical Practice. MTP Press, Lancaster, pp. 83–115
Savage M O 1984 Pathogenesis and investigation of ambiguous genitalia.
  In: Anysley-Green A (ed) Paediatric Endocrinology in Clinical Practice.
  MTP Press, Lancaster, pp. 75–81

Puberty

STAGES OF PUBERTY

Girls' breast (B) development
B1 Prepubertal
B2 Breast bud, areolar diameter increased
B3 'Mini' adult breast
B4 Nipple and areola atop the breast
B5 Mature, nipple projects, areola now part of general breast shape

Boys' genital (G) development
G1 Prepubertal, testicular volume 4 ml
G2 Enlargement of testes, and scrotum which reddens and slackens
G3 Elongation of penis, testes larger
G4 Broadening of penis, growth of glans. Testes volume 12 ml and scrotum large, dark scrotal skin
G5 Adult

Both sexes' pubic hair (PH) development
PH1 Prepubertal
PH2 A few long, downy hairs, slightly pigmented
PH3 Darker, coarser, curly hair, now spreading across the midline
PH4 Adult texture, limited to pubes
PH5 Mature, spread to medial surface of thighs
PH6 Spread up linea alba

SOME NORMAL PUBERTAL EVENTS

Girls
1. Breasts and genitals develop usually before pubic hair
2. Menarche at 13 (normal range 11–15) years at a bone age corresponding to 13–14 years
3. Peak height velocity achieves up to 10 cm per year for a time during the adolescent growth spurt at stage B2–B3

41

Boys
1. Testicular enlargement is usually the first sign. A volume of 4 ml, about a medium sized, or stuffed, olive is a good guide
2. Peak height velocity in boys is 2 years later than girls, giving 2 extra years' growth before their growth spurt, accounting for the adult height sex difference

SOME NORMAL VARIATIONS TO BE DIFFERENTIATED FROM PATHOLOGICAL CAUSES

1. Premature breast development (thelarche) from 1–2 years old
2. Premature adrenarche (pubarche), pubic or axillary hair *alone* from 7 years old
3. Gynaecomastia in boys, usually bilateral, in puberty, but remember Klinefelter's syndrome (XXY)

SOME POINTERS TO ABNORMAL PUBERTAL DEVELOPMENT

1. Precocious puberty
   (i) Boys less than 9 years old — 60% pathological
   (ii) Girls less than 8 years old — 20% pathological
2. Hirsutism alone in girls

   Precocious puberty with small testes in boys, or one testis larger than the other (Leydig cell tumour) } congenital adrenal hyperplasia, hormone secreting tumour or drug
3. No pubertal change by 13.5 years or a bone age of 14.5 years or more is due to low gonadotrophin or gonadal dysgenesis. Short stature is usually present
4. Lack of progression 2 years after onset of puberty or lack of menarche 5 years after stage B2

CAUSES OF PRECOCIOUS PUBERTY

1. Local
   (i) Thelarche
   (ii) Pubarche
2. True precocious puberty
   (i) Physiological: constitutional, familial, obesity
   (ii) Hypothalamic
       a. Injury, e.g. post-traumatic, post-infective, hydrocephalus
       b. Tumour, e.g. pineal, craniopharyngioma
       c. With skin pigmentation, e.g. tuberous sclerosis, neurofibromatosis, McCune-Albright's polyostotic fibrous dysplasia
       d. Hypothyroidism
   (iii) Gonadotrophin producing tumour, e.g. teratoma, hepatoma, chorionepithelioma

False precocious puberty (girls likely to be virilised)
1. Adrenal: congenital adrenal hyperplasia, adrenal hyperplasia, carcinoma, Cushing's disease
2. Gonadal
   (i) Leydig cell tumour of testes
   (ii) Ovarian tumours, e.g. masculinising and granulosa cell
3. Drug induced: anabolic steroids

CAUSES OF DELAYED PUBERTY

1. Physiological: constitutional delay, familial delay
2. Chronic disorders
   (i) Organic, e.g. malnutrition, Crohn's disease, coeliac, diabetes mellitus, renal failure
   (ii) Emotional, e.g. emotional deprivation, anorexia nervosa, intense exercise
3. Central with low gonadotrophins
   (i) Primary isolated deficiency or with growth hormone deficiency
   (ii) Part of syndromes, e.g. Kallman's, Frölich's, Prader-Willi, Laurence-Moon-Biedl
   (iii) Secondary to tumours, e.g. craniopharyngioma
4. Gonadal with high gonadotrophins
   (i) Girls: XO, gonadal dysgenesis, resistant ovary syndrome (see below)
   (ii) Boys: congenital anorchia, orchitis, XXY, Noonan's syndrome
5. Peripheral
   (i) Androgen insensitivity, e.g. testicular feminisation
   (ii) Enzyme deficiency in steroid biosynthesis, e.g. 17α hydoxylase

CAUSES OF PRIMARY AMENORRHOEA

1. Delayed puberty (see above)
2. Normal sexual development
   (i) Imperforate hymen
   (ii) Absent uterus in XX normal or XY testicular feminisation syndrome
   (iii) Resistant ovary syndrome (with very high levels of FSH and LH, defect in gonadotrophin receptors)
3. Heterosexual development
   (i) Androgenic steroids — iatrogenic, congenital adrenal hyperplasia, tumour, Cushing's syndrome
   (ii) XO/XY mosaic

CAUSES OF VAGINAL BLEEDING IN A CHILD

1. Trauma: accidental/non-accidental/sexual abuse
2. Menarche, e.g. precocious puberty
3. Oestrogen withdrawal
    (i) At birth
    (ii) Ingestion of contraceptive pill
4. Foreign body
5. Haemorrhagic disorders
6. Tumour: sarcoma botyroides, clear-cell adenocarcinoma (maternal diethyl stilboestrol)

CAUSES OF VAGINAL DISCHARGE

1. Physiological mucoid
2. Non-specific vaginitis; poor hygiene, tight clothing
3. Infection
   Bacterial: gonococcus, *Shigella flexneri*, pneumococcus, streptococcus
   Viral: herpes simplex
   Fungal: *Candida albicans*
   Parasites: threadworms, trichomonas
4. Foreign body
5. Tumour: adenocarcinoma etc.

CAUSES OF OLIGOMENORRHOEA

1. (i) Physiological (up to 2 years after menarche)
    (ii) Pregnancy
2. Pathological (increasingly irregular or preceded by normal menses)
    (i) Hypothalamic: stress, acute dieting, anorexia nervosa, hyperprolactinaemia, contraceptive pill, tumour
    (ii) Ovarian: polycystic ovary, gonadal dysgenesis, 47XXX, resistant ovary syndrome, tumour, premature menopause
    (iii) Adrenal: Cushing's syndrome, congenital adrenal hyperplasia, tumour
    (iv) Thyroid: hyperthyroidism

CAUSES OF MENORRHAGIA

1. Physiological
    (i) After menarche
    (ii) At ovulation (spotting)
    (iii) Abortion
2. Coagulation defects: thrombocytopenia, Von Willebrand's disease etc
3. Malignancy

FURTHER READING

Brook C G D 1978 Practical paediatric endocrinology. Academic Press, London, Ch 8
Vlies R 1985 Gynaecological problems of adolescents. In: Macfarlane J A (ed) Progress in Child Health 2. Churchill Livingstone, Edinburgh, pp. 103–117
Dewhurst J 1980 Practical pediatric and adolescent gynecology. Marcel Dekker, New York

Endocrinology

CAUSES OF GROWTH HORMONE DEFICIENCY AND HYPOPITUITARISM

Abnormality may be absence of hypothalamic releasing or inhibiting hormone, a defect in the portal system or pituitary gland.

1. Congenital
   - (i) Idiopathic: isolated or combined with gonadotrophin deficiency TSH or, rarely, ACTH
   - (ii) Pituitary dysgenesis: familial, or developmental midline defect, cleft lip and palate
   - (iii) Craniopharyngioma
2. Acquired
   - (i) Trauma
       - a. Birth, e.g. first-born breech
       - b. Fracture of sphenoid
   - (ii) Radiation: antileukaemia therapy
   - (iii) Other tumours: pituitary adenoma, pinealoma, optic chiasma glioma
   - (iv) TB meningitis
   - (v) Hand-Schüller-Christian disease (Histiocytosis X)
3. Partial or transient

CAUSE FOR SUSPICION OF GROWTH HORMONE DEFICIENCY

1. Symptomatic hypoglycaemia
2. Growth failure noted by 2 years old, growth velocity < 5 cm per year
3. Overweight for height from reduced gluconeogenesis
4. Immature facial features, dental malocclusion
5. Associated panhypopituitarism, e.g. hypothyroidism, hypoplastic genitals

CAUSES OF DIABETES INSIPIDUS

1. Neurogenic: antidiuretic hormone deficient
   (i) Primary idiopathic: familial
   (ii) Secondary to neurohypophyseal tract damage
      Trauma
      Infection: tuberculosis
      Tumour: craniopharyngioma, pinealoma, adenoma
      Infiltration: Hand-Schüller-Christian, leukaemias
2. Nephrogenic: antidiuretic hormone resistant, familial X-linked

CAUSES OF INAPPROPRIATE ANTIDIURETIC HORMONE SECRETION

The urinary osmolality is inappropriately high for the osmolality of serum, with normal renal and adrenal function
1. Infection: meningitis, encephalitis, Guillain-Barré
2. Stress: surgery
3. Neurogenic
   (i) Asphyxia e.g. birth or prolonged seizures
   (ii) Brain tumour, porphyria
4. Respiratory: bronchopneumonia, status asthmaticus, chronic pulmonary disease, mechanical ventilation
5. Drugs, e.g. vincristine

CAUSES OF HYPOTHYROIDISM

1. Non-goitrous
   (i) Congenital: athyreosis, hypoplasia (may present as 'late' failure), ectopic
   (ii) Secondary to hypothalamic (↓ TRH) or pituitary (↓ TSH) defect: isolated defect of TRH or TSH, trauma, infection, infiltration, tumours, dysgenesis
2. Goitrous
   (i) Neonatal
      a. Familial dyshormonogenesis. Defect in iodine trapping, organification of iodine (+ deafness = Pendred's syndrome), iodotyrosine coupling, iodotyrosine deiodination, abnormal thyroglobulins
      b. Maternal goitrogens
   (ii) Childhood
      a. Autoimmune thyroiditis
      b. Endemic hypothyroidism (iodine deficiency)
      c. Familial dyshormonogenesis
      d. Drugs e.g. sulphonamides, phenylbutazone, PAS, resorcinol, cobalt

CONDITIONS COMMONLY CONFUSED WITH DIABETES MELLITUS

1. Glycosuria present
    (i) Convulsions
    (ii) Chemical diabetes in acute infections
    (iii) Renal glycosuria
    (iv) Salicylate poisoning
    (v) Hypernatraemic dehydration
    (vi) Acute pancreatitis
    (vii) Other causes of glycosuria
        a. CNS infection, trauma, tumour, haemorrhage
        b. Cushing's disease
        c. Lead poisoning
        d. Fanconi's syndrome
2. Glycosuria absent
    (i) Acute infections, e.g. pneumonia, urinary tract infection, meningitis
    (ii) Acute abdomen
    (iii) Diabetes insipidus
    (iv) Compulsive drinking

CAUSES OF HYPOGLYCAEMIA

Neonatal hypoglycaemia (see p. 23)

Older ages
1. Decreased substrate
    (i) Malnutrition
    (ii) Accelerated starvation (ketotic hypoglycaemia)
    (iii) Stress, e.g. septicaemia, hypothermia etc
2. Drugs: alcohol, antihistamines, ackee nut, diguanides and sulphonylureas, salicylates
3. Hepatic damage
    (i) Acute liver disease, e.g. hepatitis
    (ii) Reye's syndrome
    (iii) Maple syrup urine disease
4. Endocrine
    (i) Hyperinsulinism, e.g. hyperplasia, tumour
    (ii) Hypopituitarism, hypothyroidism, hypoadrenalism
5. Decreased hepatic release due to enzyme deficiencies
    (i) Glycogenoses: von Gierkes, debrancher enzyme (p. 152)
    (ii) Fructose 1: 6 diphosphatase
    (iii) Galactosaemia, fructosaemia

CAUSES OF OBESITY

1. Exogenous: often familial, usually tall for age, advanced bone age

2. Pathological: usually sporadic, short stature, bone age normal
   or delayed
   (i) Endocrine: hypothyroidism, Cushing's syndrome
   (ii) Tumour: Fröhlich's hypothalamic tumour
   (iii) Genetic: Laurence-Moon-Biedl, Prader-Willi

SIDE EFFECTS OF SYSTEMIC GLUCOCORTICOID ADMINISTRATION

1. Catabolic: short stature, osteoporosis, bone age retarded, striae, ecchymoses, muscular weakness
2. Gluconeogenesis: cushingoid facies, trunkal obesity, buffalo hump, hyperglycaemia, diabetes mellitus
3. Cortisol excess: water and salt retention, hypokalaemia metabolic alkalosis, hypertension, headaches, hypercalciuria, renal calculi
4. Androgenic: hirsutism, acne, amenorrhoea
5. Neurological: emotional lability, raised intracranial pressure, epileptic tendency
6. Immunosuppression: infections, e.g. TB, candida, chickenpox
7. Adrenal suppression and atrophy
8. Gastrointestinal: gastric irritation, peptic ulceration and perforation, pancreatitis
9. Polycythaemia
10. Withdrawal: vomiting, hypercalcaemia, rebound of disease

ADDITIONAL FEATURES SEEN IN CUSHING'S SYNDROME

1. Virilisation, advanced skeletal age and rapid growth occasionally
2. Hyperpigmentation from excess adrenocorticotrophic hormone

CAUSES OF ADRENAL INSUFFICIENCY

Neonatal
1. Haemorrhage from asphyxia, shock, septicaemia
2. Congenital adrenal hyperplasia
3. Congenital adrenal hypoplasia, alone/anencephaly, maternal steroid administration

Later
1. Glucocorticoid withdrawal, therapeutic or surgical
2. Waterhouse-Friedrichsen syndrome
3. Congenital adrenal hyperplasia
4. Hypopituitarism
5. Addison's disease ± mucocutaneous candidiasis

CONGENITAL ADRENAL HYPERPLASIA

Incidence about 1 in 5000, 90% as 21-hydroxylase defect (4 below).
Simplified outline of synthesis:

```
              cholesterol
                1 ↓
              pregnanelone
                2 ↓
        4                    3
DOCA  ←  progesterone  →  17-hydroxy progesterone
5 ↓                    4 ↓                    ↓ 2
ALDOSTERONE      11-deoxycortisol        androstenedione
                      5 ↓                    ↓
                   CORTISOL            TESTOSTERONE
```

CLINICAL FEATURES

Enzyme deficiency	Ambiguous genitalia	Female virilisation	Salt loss	Hypertension from DOCA
1. 20.22 Desmolase	Males	−		
2. 3β hydroxysteroid dehydrogenase	Males	+	+	
3. 17α hydroxylase	Males	−	+	+
4. 21 α hydroxylase	Females	+	in 50%	
5. 11β hydroxylase	Females	+	−	+

1–3 = Reduced testosterone synthesis
4, 5 = Excessive androgen production

Neurology

NORMAL VARIATIONS

1. Plagiocephaly (skull asymmetry caused by intrauterine moulding and later by lying mainly on one side). Also in severe hypotonia, cerebral palsy, craniostenosis, sternomastoid tumour
2. Fontanelle closure
   Posterior fontanelle by 1–6 weeks
   Anterior fontanelle by 18–24 months
3. Eyes
   (i) Structure
      a. Size at birth: two-thirds adult, corneal diameter similar to adult
      b. Apparent squint (common in infancy) from a relatively lateral inner canthus of the eye. A true squint is excluded if a light shone at the eyes is reflected off the same spot on each pupil (see p. 56)
      c. Optic disc: pale, later becomes pink. Optic atrophy may be difficult to detect
   (ii) Function
      a. 'Setting sun' sign: physiological at 2–4 months old
      b. Vision: present at birth, acuity achieves adult levels by 1 year

A BASIC NEUROLOGICAL EXAMINATION

A. OBSERVATION

1. Activities
   (i) Speech, play, manipulation and coordination of hands in handling pencil, toy bricks, dolls etc in age appropriate way

SOME MILESTONES IN NORMAL DEVELOPMENT
Know at least one item per category for each age band

Social	Hearing and speech	Vision and fine motor	Gross motor
6 weeks			
1. Smiles (H) 2. Coos (H)	1. Stills to mother's voice or toy bell	1. Follows face in 90° arc 2. Stares intently	1. Sat up: lifts head few seconds 2. Examiner's hand lifting from under the body: head in line with the trunk 3. Primitive reflexes (p. 12) present
6 to 9 months			6 months:
1. Objects go to mouth 2. Enjoys bath and 'bool!' (H) 3. No longer looks at hand; looks at foot 4. Chews on biscuit (H)	1. 6 months: 'ma,da' 2. 9 months: babbles, 'Mama, dada', understands 'no-no', 'bye-bye' (H) 3. Responds to own name 4. Hearing test (p. 59)	1. Cover test (p. 56) 2. Eyes fix on pellet of paper 3. At 6 months forgets falling object; by 9 months follows it 4. 6 months: palmar grasp; 7 months: transfers; 9 months: index finger probing approach	1. Rolls from back to front 2. Sits alone few seconds 3. Flexes head and trunk when pulled to sit 9 months: 1. Sits securely 2. Pulls up on furniture to stand
One year			
1. Comes when called 2. Lets go on request; finds hidden item	1. Shakes head for 'no' 2. Understands some words; says 1 to 3 words (H)	1. Picks up crumbs with pincer grasp 2. Throws toys deliberately, watching fall	1. Pivots when sitting 2. Walks alone or one hand held

H = by history, objective enough for most cases; otherwise by direct observation

Social	Hearing and speech	Vision and fine motor	Gross motor
3. Dress; cooperates, pushing arm through sleeve		to ground 3. Holds 1 inch cube in each hand, bangs together, may make 2 cube high tower	
18 months 1. Cup: lifts, drinks and puts down (H) 2. Spoon: feeds self (H) 3. Toilet: bowels – clean. Wet nappy discarded (H) 4. Copies: dusting, washing up, sweeping (H)	1. Jargons++ 2. Points to 3 parts of body 3. Obeys single command 'get your cup', etc 4. Says 6 words; Echolalia	1. Fisted grasp of pencil, scribbles 2. Points at wants 3. Picks up threads, pins, etc, neatly 4. Turns pages in picture book, 2 at a time 5. Tower of 3–4 × 1 inch cubes	1. Walks well 2. Throws toy without falling 3. Climbs stairs (H)
2 to 2½ years 1. Toilet: dry reliably by day, and tells in time (H) 2. No sharing, plays alone, tantrums (H), demanding (H) 3. Imaginative play	1. Many words 2. Phrase of 2–3 words (H) 3. Knows name 4. Understands 'give dolly a drink', i.e. has inner language	1. Drawing: imitates vertical and horizontal line and circle 2. Tower: 6–8 cubes 3. Book: turns one page at a time	1. Runs 2. Kicks ball 3. Jumps on the spot 4. Stairs: 2 feet per tread 5. Trike: pushes with feet
3 to 3½ years 1. Toilet: pulls pants down and up alone (H) 2. Eating: fork and spoon together (H)	1. Gives full name, sex 2. Counts by rote to 10 3. Uses 'me', 'I', 'you'	1. Colour matches 2+ colours correctly 2. Mature pencil grip; copies circle	1. Stands on one leg momentarily 2. Stairs; adult style of ascent (H)

Social	Hearing and speech	Vision and fine motor	Gross motor
3. Plays with other child, shares toy (H)	4. Understands on, under, back of, etc	3. Identifies square, triangle, although cannot draw them	3. Trike: pedals (H)
4 to 5 years			
1. Toilet: wipes own bottom (H)	1. Gives name, address, age	1. Colours: matches 4+	1. Hops
2. Eating: knife and fork (H)	2. Counts to 10	2. Drawing: 4 years copies cross and square, by 5 years a triangle, draws a man with head, arms, legs and fingers	2. Climbs trees (H)
3. Dress: on and off unsupervised except tie, laces (H)	3. Grammar OK		3. Ball games, 'catch', etc (H)
4. Plays by the rules, competitive	4. Articulation almost mature		

    (ii) Awareness: altered by seizures, drugs, hypoglycaemia etc
       (p. 69)
2. Locomotion: crawl or gait asymmetrical or abnormal, listening
   for foot fall. Pseudoparesis if acutely painful e.g. osteomyelitis,
   trauma etc
    (i) Limp (p. 158): hemiplegia, joint disease
    (ii) Broad based gait: ataxia (p. 70), dyskinetic cerebral palsy
       (CP)
    (iii) Tip-toe: CP with scissoring of legs, muscular dystrophy,
       polyneuritis
    (iv) Waddling gait: congenital dislocation hip, Duchênne
       muscular dystrophy, polymyositis, old polio peripheral
       neuropathy
    (v) Foot drop: sciatic nerve damage, perineal muscular atrophy,
       heavy metal poisoning
    (iv) Pes cavus: Friedreich's ataxia, spinal cord lesions

B. EXAMINATION OF CRANIAL NERVES

1. Developmental abilities: selected items for the pre-school child
   (see above, pp. 52–54). At school age try reading and the four
   mathematical functions $(+, -, \times, \div)$, writing name, age, address
   etc as appropriate
2. Cranial nerves: smell, vision, eye movements, corneal, facial,
   hearing, bulbar, accessory (see below)

SMELL
Usually obtained on history

VISION

Visual fields
Infant: sat on a lap facing you, attention obtained by your holding an object with one hand while the other brings in another object in each of the 4 quadrants in turn. Look for his fixation of the second object. A homonomous hemianopia can be detected, but a bitemporal hemianopia needs each eye to be covered separately and may be resisted vigorously

Older child: confrontation, with you about half a metre away, both arms abducted, facing the child who is told to look at your nose. He/she should point to the index finger that is wiggled.

Each eye is then covered in turn, his right and your left by the individual's own respective hand, and, with your arm extended to the limits of the visual field in each quadrant, each wiggle is affirmed by his responding 'yes'. Repeat the wiggle to confirm recognition of the signal

Ophthalmoscopy
Examine with ophthalmoscope, cornea and lens (p. 9), media and retina usually towards the end of assessment

EYE MOVEMENTS

Encourage visual pursuit of a finger or object. The infant and toddler usually needs to have his/her head held still in the midline by a restraining hand
1. Look for ptosis, pupil size (smaller on side with Horner's syndrome), nystagmus (p. 70)
2. Conjugate eye deviation:
   Downwards (sunsetting): in raised intracranial pressure, kernicterus, some normal infants
   To one side: 'looking at' — an acute irritative lesion in the frontal lobe (destructive or seizure)
      'away' — from old lesion (hemiplegia)
3. Third nerve lesion shows ptosis, dilated pupil and lateral deviation on the affected side
4. Sixth nerve lesion causes medial deviation of the affected side. If facial palsy also present a brain stem lesion is likely, otherwise may be false localising sign of raised intracranial pressure
5. Head tilt to one side may be to compensate for a verical squint. *Beware* posterior fossa tumour
6. Corneal light reflex: refletion of ophthalmoscope light is in the same spot on each eye. Overcomes the problem of apparent

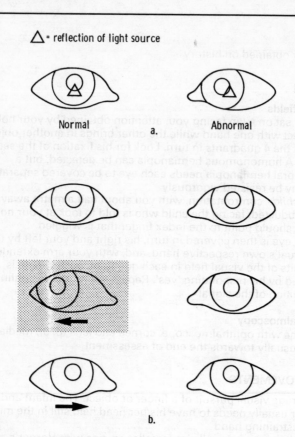

△ = reflection of light source

Normal   Abnormal

a.

b.

Fig. 6

squint due to a broad nasal bridge. Figure 6a shows abnormal reflection

7. Cover test:
   Cover each eye in turn using a card, parent's hand, or examiner's thumb swinging from one eye to the other with other fingers resting gently on crown of baby's head. Then use a toy, keys or light to attract attention, holding the toy/keys at 30 cm, and repeat at 2 m.

   A latent squint is detected when the affected eye turns in or out, returning to its original position on being uncovered, as in Figure 6b.

   In manifest squint the squinting eye will fix when the other eye is covered, and move back when uncovered. In alternating squint either eye squints on covering.

N.B. Resentment to covering one eye (the good one) may indicate abnormality in the other

Causes of squint

1. Non-paralytic (concomitant)
   (i) Failure of fusion of images (often inherited)
   (ii) Lens abnormalities (refractive errors, cataract)
   (iii) Nerve weakness due to febrile illness, head injury, cerebral palsy
   (iv) Retinal: retrolental fibroplasia, optic atrophy, detachment (trauma), scar (congenital infection)
2. Paralytic (incomitant):
   (i) Congenital: cranial nerve agenesis
   (ii) Tumour, false localising sign in raised intracranial pressure

Causes of blindness and partial sight

1. Eye: retrolental fibroplasia, retinal detachment, trauma, cataracts (p. 73), optic atrophy, retinal degenerations, malformation, ophthalmia neonatorum, acute exanthema, hypovitaminosis A, retinoblastoma
2. Optic nerve or its radiation: tumour, trauma
3. Cortical: damage to the occipital cortex and its connections owing to trauma, meningitis, birth asphyxia, hydrocephalus

Causes of amblyopia

Amblyopia: reduced visual acuity in one eye compared with the other, which if severe and uncorrected may result in permanent visual impairment
1. Structural: corneal opacity, cataract, ptosis
2. Blurred image: refractive error, albinism
3. Squint (p. 57)

Timing and nature of vision testing

Newborn: direct observation of eyes for abnormality, testing for the red reflex using an ophthalmoscope (p. 9)

6 Weeks: history and mother's comments. Look for persistent squints (abnormal at any age), abnormal eye movements, lack of visual fixation of the face (delayed maturation, blind, autistic)

6 Months: any squint refer to eye specialist, check eyes with ophthalmoscope, do cover test for near and far vision

4 Years: (i) Letter or symbol matching test e.g. Sheridan-Gardiner 5 or 7 letter test
(ii) Cover test
(iii) Stereoscopic vision test (Random dot stereogram)

8 Years: colour vision testing (Ishihara)

The snellen letter chart for distant vision

6/6   =   Normal vision, identifies correctly at 6 m
6/5   =   Superior vision
6/18 =   Moderately poor, sees at 6 m that normally seen from
          18 m away
6/60 =   Poor visual acuity

Reduced Snellen chart is used for near vision or type size where normal visual acuity = N5

CORNEAL (fifth sensory) reflex

Whisp of cotton wool is traditional. Better tolerated: gently blow at the eyes, and a blink is readily elicited in the conscious person

FACIAL (seventh)

Crying, baring teeth or laughing elicits asymmetry. Puffing out the cheeks and burying eyelashes ('close eyes tight') is impaired in myopathies

Causes of facial palsy

A. Upper motor neurone lesion (upper half of face moves)
1. Cerebral palsy: hemiplegia, tetraplegia
2. Cerebral cortex tumour

B. Lower motor neurone lesion (eyelid may not close, brow not wrinkle)
Acquired
1. Infection
    (i) In middle ear, mastoid
    (ii) Encephalitis
    (iii) Guillain-Barré syndrome
2. Trauma
3. Idiopathic (Bell's palsy)
4. Hypertension
5. Brain stem tumour, leukaemia deposit
Congenital
Nuclear agenesis: Moebius' syndrome (usually with 6th nerve weakness bilaterally)

C. Myopathies: dystrophia myotonica, congenital myopathies

HEARING TESTS

1. Infancy
   Present quiet noises made with cup and spoon, rustling paper, high pitched rattle, whispered 's', 'oo' and baby's name. The head or eyes should turn to the side tested
   7 months at 50 cm from ear and 45° behind baby's ear
   9 months at 1 m from ear, 45° behind baby's ear and level with it
2. Pre-school 2½–3 year old
   (i) Identifying objects: points to common objects the names of which have already been said, then repeated at quieter sound levels during the test
   (ii) 'Go' and 'sss' games: conditioning the child to place an object (toy) in a box each time you say 'go' or 'sss' at successively quieter sound levels
   (iii) Tuning fork tests
       a. Air–bone conduction (Rinne test): if the sound is better transmitted via bone, (place tuning fork on mastoid as soon as child indicates sound no longer heard at external ear) then middle ear fluid should be suspected
       b. Confirmation of unilateral impairment by the Weber test: tuning fork on forehead localises sound better to affected side in middle ear problem, and to the normal side in nerve deafness. Not helpful in bilateral disease

Causes of deafness/failed hearing-test

1. Acute otitis media ⎫
2. Serous otitis media ⎬ conductive deafness
3. Congenital ⎭
   (i) Genetic, unknown — conductive plus nerve deafness
   (ii) Infection, e.g. rubella, cytomegalovirus → nerve deafness
4. Perinatal: asphyxia, hyperbilirubinaemia, drugs, prematurity — nerve deafness

BULBAR NERVES

Nasal or 'cleft palate' speech, poor palatal movement on testing for gag (last test of all!) in 9th and 10th nerve lesions. Tongue deviates to the affected side when stuck out — 12th nerve

Causes of bulbar weakness

1. Cerebral palsy (supra-bulbar origin)
2. Infection/parainfection: encephalitis, polio, tetanus, diphtheria, TB, meningitis, Guillain-Barré syndrome, rabies, botulism
3. Drugs: phenothiazines, metoclopramide
4. Brain stem tumour

5. Rare: myasthenia gravis, dystrophia myotonica, Möebius'
   syndrome of cranial nerve agenesis, Gaucher's disease,
   Pompe's disease
N.B. Acute onset of drooling is a symptom of stomatitis,
pharyngitis or epiglottitis

ACCESSORY NERVE

Trapezius and sternomastoid weakness on hunching shoulders and
turning head towards a toy, due to cerebral palsy, Guillain-Barré
syndrome, tumour of brain stem

C. SENSORY

In the infant, reaction to cotton wool or a pin may be indicated in
brachial nerve palsy, and spina bifida to establish the extent and
level of the lesion. Older children can be tested conventionally

D. MOTOR

Observation of spontaneous movement is a continuous process
during the examination, as in A.
   Tone is influenced by neck posture (p. 12). It is not to be
confused with power or ligamentous laxity. Infants who appear
flexed and hypertonic when prone may show themselves to be
quite floppy when pulled up from lying supine into the sitting
position. See pp. 12, 71 for causes of floppy infants.
   Hypertonic infants show fisting, thumbs tucked into palms; when
reaching they are clumsy, often having a 'rake' like grasp long past
the expected time for its disappearance. The older child may show
fixed flexion deformities due to immobility. See p. 68 for causes of
cerebral palsy.
   Variability in tone of the limbs is a hallmark of athetosis. Affected
infants may be very floppy.
   Coordination is assessed in the infant by picking up a pellet of
paper; in the pre-school child by building bricks, play at feeding
dolls, threading beads; in the older child by rapid sequential finger
— thumb apposition, finger — nose, heel–toe walking etc. For
causes of ataxia see p. 70.
   For causes of repetitive movements see p. 75

E. REFLEXES

The deep tendon jerks (DTJs) are brisker in neonates than older
infants, who often have easily elicited knee jerks (tap the front of
the tibia, starting at the ankle). Relatively sluggish in the upper
limbs compared with adults. Maintain the head in the midline to
avoid the influence of the asymmetric tonic reflex

CAUSES OF ABNORMAL DEEP TENDON JERKS

A. Increased
1. Decerebration with rigidity of tone: asphyxia, raised intracranial pressure (blood, CSF, encephalitis, tumour)
2. Cerebral palsy
3. Hysteria
4. Degenerative encephalopathies (p. 62)
5. Spinal lesion (below the lesion)

B. Diminished
1. Central: drugs, Down's syndrome, mental retardation, cerebellar lesions (p. 70)
2. Spinal: polio, spinal muscular atrophy
3. Peripheral neuropathy: Friedreich's ataxia, Guillain-Barré, heavy metal poisoning
4. Neuromuscular junction: myasthenia gravis
5. Muscular weakness: Duchênne, etc

Cutaneous reflexes
Abdominal (T7–12) and cremasteric (L1) reflexes present from 4 months, the plantar reflex (S1) is initially flexor in the first week becoming extensor until walking is achieved. Use a thumb nail and stroke the outer border of the foot to avoid eliciting a plantar grasp reflex. The anal reflex (S4,5) is present from birth, and 'winking' is obtained by firm stroking with a thin wooden stick perianally.

Useful in recent hemiplegias, spinal cord lesions, sphincter problems.

F. SKIN, HEAD CIRCUMFERENCE (p. 72)

If not already looked for, check for café au lait patches and axillary freckling of neurofibromatosis, ash leaf shaped pale lesions of tuberous sclerosis

DEVELOPMENTAL WARNING SIGNS

1. At any age
   (i) Family history of note, e.g. deafness, cataracts
   (ii) Maternal concern
   (iii) Dribbling incontinence
   (iv) Persistent obligatory asymmetric tonic neck reflex
   (v) Persistent squint
   (vi) Discordance in developmental abilities in different areas
   (vii) Regression in previously acquired skills
2. At 6 months
   (i) Persistent primitive reflexes (Moro, stepping, palmar grasp, asymmetric tonic neck reflex)

   (ii) Squint, intermittent or persistent
   (iii) Hand preference, e.g. hemiplegia
   (iv) Little interest in noises, people, playthings (average 3–4
        months)
3. At 10–12 months
   (i) Not sitting unsupported for 10 minutes (average 9 months)
   (ii) No double syllable babble, e.g. 'Baba', 'Dada' (average 8
        months)
   (iii) Lack of sustained visual interest (average 9 months)
4. At 18 months
   (i) Not walking independently (average 15 months). In a boy
        consider Duchenne muscular dystrophy, *in either sex*
        congenital dislocation of the hip
   (ii) Less than 6 words other than mama, baba, dada (average
        15 months)
   (iii) Persistent mouthing and drooling (average 12 months)
5. At 2½ years: no 2 to 3 word sentence (average 2 years)
6. At 4 years: speech unintelligible (average 3–3½ years)

CAUSES OF DELAYED DEVELOPMENT

By and large prematurity should be taken into account when
assessing developmental progress i.e. a 3 month premature infant
at 6 months old will be at least at a 3 month level of ability, usually
more
1. Idiopathic: constitutional, familial (affecting *one* field e.g.
   bottom shuffler, catching up later)
2. Deprivation
3. Mental retardation
4. Specific abnormality e.g. blind, deaf, cerebral palsy

CAUSES OF ARRESTED OR DETERIORATING DEVELOPMENT

1. Emotional deprivation
2. Intercurrent illness, e.g. malabsorption
3. Acute cerebral injury, e.g. encephalitis, trauma
4. Seizures: uncontrolled, prolonged
5. Drugs, e.g. phenytoin excess
6. Hydrocephalus
7. Metabolic, e.g. hypothyroidism, lead poisoning
8. Degenerations
   (i) Infections: AIDS, subacute sclerosing panencephalitis
   (ii) Genetic: Wilson's disease, Huntington's chorea, lysosomal
        storage disorders (pp. 153, 154)

CAUSES OF MENTAL HANDICAP

1. Idiopathic
2. Prenatal
   (i) Genetic:
      a. chromosomal e.g. Down's syndrome, X linked mental retardation (p. 3), XO
      b. familial e.g. tuberous sclerosis, inborn errors of metabolism
   (ii) Congenital infection: TORCH p. 2
   (iii) Alcohol; drugs e.g. phenytoin
3. Perinatal: asphyxia, birth injury, prematurity
4. Postnatal: meningitis, head injury (accidental and non-accidental), prolonged seizures, lead poisoning, hypothyroidism

CAUSES OF OVERACTIVE BEHAVIOUR

1. Organic
   (i) Mental retardation
   (ii) Epilepsy
   (iii) Phenobarbitone
   (iv) Hyperkinetic syndrome?
2. Psychiatric
3. Educational
   (i) Specific learning difficulties
   (ii) Inappropriate educational, social or cultural match
4. Individual 'high drive'

CAUSES OF 'AUTISTIC' BEHAVIOUR

1. Mental retardation
2. Overactive behaviour
3. Epilepsy
4. Cerebral palsy
5. Sensory deficit: deafness, blindness
6. Aphasia
7. Autism (onset by 2 years, delayed speech, emotional impairment, odd repetitive movements, resistance to change, inappropriate anxiety or rage, unexpected abilities)

CAUSES OF RETARDED SPEECH

1. Deprivation
2. Developmental delay in speech
3. Deaf
4. Delayed mental development
5. Deranged, e.g. autism
6. Dementing: degenerative diseases (p. 62)
7. Dumb: elective mutism

Normal lumbar CSF values

Age	WBC × 10^6/l	RBC × 10^6/l	Glucose mmol/l	Protein g/l
Premature	0–100	0–1000		0.4–3.0
			1.0–4.0	
Term	0–14	50–800		0.3–1.0
Infant/child	0–5	0–2	2.8–4.4	0.1–0.4

CAUSES OF CSF LYMPHOCYTOSIS

1. Normal CSF glucose
   (i) Viral
   (ii) Leptospirosis
   (iii) Cryptococcus
   (iv) Kawasaki disease
2. CSF glucose usually less than two thirds' blood sugar
   (i) Partially treated bacterial meningitis
   (ii) TB meningitis
   (iii) Cerebral abscess
   (iv) Leukaemia

Organisms found in bacterial meningitis

Age	Common	Less common
Newborn to 6 months	Gram negative: Escherichia coli Gram positive: Staphylococcus aureus, epidermidis (congenital CNS abnormalities, valves etc)	Proteus vulgaris Pseudomonas Group B streptococcus Listeria monocytogenes
Older ages	Gram negative: Neisseria meningitidis Haemophilus influenzae Gram positive: Streptococcus pneumoniae	Klebsiella, salmonella, shigella Acid and alcohol fast Mycobacterium tuberculosis

Causes of recurrence of fever in treated meningitis

1. Phlebitis
2. Unknown
3. Drug fever
4. Viral infection
5. Urinary tract infection
6. Resistant organism, inadequate or inappropriate antibiotic
7. Commonly sought, rarely found: abscess, large effusion, otitis media

CAUSES OF NEONATAL SEIZURES

1. In the first 2 days of life
   (i) Hypoxic — ischaemic encephalopathy
   (ii) Birth injury
   (iii) Intracranial haemorrhage
   (iv) Metabolic: hypoglycaemia, stress hypocalcaemia (normal phosphate), hyponatraemia, pyridoxine dependency
   (v) Drug withdrawal
   (vi) Brain cortex dysplasia
2. Age 1 week
   (i) Metabolic: hypocalcaemia (elevated phosphate), hypomagnesaemia, kernicterus, amino aciduria, galactosaemia, hypernatraemia, hexachlorophane poisoning
   (ii) Infection
      a. Congenital: toxoplasma, other, rubella, cytomegalovirus, Herpes simplex (TORCH)
      b. Acquired: bacterial, e.g. Gram negative, group B streptococcus
   (iii) Genetic: familial neonatal fits, tuberous sclerosis etc
   (iv) Idiopathic: '5th day fits'

Seizures by age

Type	Age	Clinical/EEG
Neonatal	0–4 weeks	Tonic in premature, asphyxia, clonic in term infants
Infantile spasms	3–9 months	Lightning jerks or nods. EEG: hypsarrhythmia
Lennox-Gastaut	2–7 years	Absence, myoclonic jerks, nocturnal fits. EEG $2\frac{1}{2}$–4s spike and wave
Febrile convulsion	6 months –5 years	Generalised or focal fit. EEG normal
Petit mal	3–15 years	Classical absence of 15–30s. EEG: 3/s spike and wave
Benign focal epilepsy of childhood	7–10 years	Tongue sensations, focal → generalised fit. EEG: Rolandic spikes, not midtemporal
Massive myoclonus (rare)	9–14 years	On waking, mainly girls at menstruation. EEG: atypical spike, polyspike
Photosensitive	8–14 years	Flicker induced fit and spike and wave on EEG
Grand mal	Any age Peak 6–10 years	Tonic and/or clonic, no aura. EEG: bilateral abnormality
Temporal lobe	Any age Peak 5–7 years	Aura, tonic-clonic, automatisms. EEG: focal abnormality

CAUSES OF SEIZURES BETWEEN 1 AND 6 MONTHS

1. Infection
    (i) Bacterial meningitis: Gram negative organisms (p. 64)
    (ii) Viral meningitis: Herpes simplex, chickenpox
    (iii) Congenital: TORCH
2. Trauma: non-accidental injury, chronic subdurals
3. Metabolic
    (i) Hypoglycaemia (p. 48)
    (ii) Hypernatraemia
    (iii) Hypocalcaemia e.g. rickets, hypoparathyroidism
    (iv) Inborn errors e.g. amino aciduria, glycogen storage, neurolipidoses, Menke's kinky hair syndrome
4. Structural e.g. cerebral palsy, congenital malformations
5. Idiopathic e.g. cryptogenic infantile spasms (p. 66), idiopathic epilepsy
6. Miscellaneous: haemolytic uraemic syndrome (p. 183), Reye's syndrome (p. 184), post-immunisation

Causes of infantile spasms, and Lennox-Gastaut syndrome of absences, seizures of akinetic, nocturnal, jacknife and massive myoclonic type usually with mental retardation
1. Cryptogenic
2. Infection
    (i) Congenital e.g. TORCH (p. 2), syphilis
    (ii) Encephalitis, meningitis
3. Perinatal, e.g. prematurity, asphyxia, birth injury
4. Congenital abnormalities e.g. hydranencephaly, porencephaly, absent corpus callosum, agyria
5. Non-accidental injury
6. Tuberous sclerosis
7. Metabolic e.g. hypoglycaemia, PKU, lipidoses (p. 153).
8. Post-pertussis immunisation?

CAUSES OF SEIZURES AFTER EARLY INFANCY

1. Febrile convulsions
2. Epilepsy
3. Structural: cerebral palsy, post-traumatic, perinatal injury
4. Infection
    (i) Bacterial meningitis: meningococcus, *Haemophilus influenzae*, pneumococcus, tuberculosis
    (ii) Viral: exanthema, Herpes simplex, slow virus (e.g. SSPE, AIDS), immunisation
5. Parainfective: immunisation, Reye's syndrome
6. Toxins
    (i) Drugs, e.g. salicylates, alcohol
    (ii) Heavy metals e.g. lead, cadmium
    (iii) Scalds

7. Metabolic (see above)
8. Tumour, cerebral leukaemia
9. Vascular: arterio-venous malformation, intracranial haemorrhage, carotid arteritis in HHE syndrome (hyperpyrexia, hemiplegia, epilepsy)

CAUSES OF FOCAL SEIZURES

1. Febrile convulsions
2. Idiopathic (commonest of apyrexial seizures)
3. Cerebral scar
   (i) Prolonged febrile convulsion
   (ii) Infection
   (iii) Birth injury, trauma
4. Temporal lobe epilepsy
5. Space occupation: tumour, abscess, cyst (all rare causes)
6. Congenital: arteriovenous malformations, hamartomas

CAUSES OF CONDITIONS COMMONLY MISTAKEN FOR EPILEPSY

1. Delirium, rigors e.g. fever, drugs, alcohol
2. Sleep related
   (i) Night terrors, sleep walking, enuresis
   (ii) Sleep startles in neonates, jerks in older children
   (iii) Narcolepsy
3. Cerebral ischaemia
   (i) Syncopy
   (ii) Breath holding attacks
   (iii) Hyperventilation, 'fainting lark', severe asthma
   (iv) Stokes-Adams attacks
4. Behavioural e.g. ritualistic pre-sleep behaviour, masturbation, tics, panic attacks
5. Migraine, periodic syndrome
6. Vertigo
   (i) Drugs, alcohol
   (ii) Benign paroxysmal vertigo
   (iii) Vestibular neuronitis
7. Hypoglycaemia (p. 48)
8. Involuntary movements e.g. chorea
9. Munchausen by proxy

CAUSES OF UNCONTROLLED EPILEPSY

1. Non-compliance or inadequate medication
2. Intoxication by drug excess or idiosyncratic response
3. Wrong drug
4. Liver enzyme induction
5. Psychological stress
6. Structural abnormality e.g. hydrocephalus, tuberous sclerosis

7. Tumour
8. Degeneration e.g. Tay-Sach's, Batten's, subacute sclerosing panencephalitis

CAUSES OF HEADACHE

1. Tension, especially likely in school refusal (p. 75)
2. Migraine
3. Raised intracranial pressure: tumour, abscess
4. Post-traumatic
5. Infection: meningitis
6. Sinusitis, dental caries
7. Hypertension (rare)
8. Intracranial bleed (rare)

COMMON CAUSES OF CEREBRAL PALSY

1. Hemiplegia
   (i)   Birth injury, non-accidental injury
   (ii) Congenital
   (iii) Causes of acute hemiplegia
2. Double hemiplegia: congenital, birth asphyxia, cardiac arrest, CNS infections
3. Diplegia: prematurity, familial
4. Ataxia: congenital, trauma, infection
5. Ataxic diplegia: hydrocephalus
6. Athetoid: birth asphyxia, kernicterus, cardiac arrest

Causes of acute hemiplegia

1. Unknown
2. Cerebral arteritis: upper respiratory tract infections and cervical adenitis common
3. Trauma: cerebral, carotid artery, bone fracture with fat embolism
4. Infection: encephalitis e.g. herpes simplex
5. Parainfection: exanthema (measles, chickenpox), post-immunisation
6. Arteriovenous malformations
8. Cardiac: hyperviscocity in cyanotic lesions, embolism, bacterial endocarditis, atrial myxoma (rare)
9. Haematological
   (i) Bleeding, e.g. idiopathic thrombocytopenia, leukaemia, haemophilia
   (ii) Sickle cell

10. Miscellaneous
     (i) Dehydration; sinus thrombosis, hypernatraemia
     (ii) Homocystinuria
     (iii) Connective tissue e.g. polyarteritis nodosa
     (iv) Moya moya disease of telangiectasia of cerebral blood
          vessels

CAUSES OF COMA

1. Primary CNS abnormality
     (i) Epilepsy
     (ii) Trauma: accidental, non-accidental
     (iii) Infection: meningitis, encephalitis
     (iv) Parainfection: exanthema, post-vaccination, Reye's
          syndrome of coma, fatty liver, hypoglycaemia, acidaemia
     (v) Vascular: thrombosis, haemorrhage, embolism
     (vi) Tumour: cerebral leukaemia
     (vii) Degeneration of central nervous system
2. Exogenous poisons
     (i) Drugs
          a. Accidental: tricyclics, benzodiazepines, iron, salicylates,
             barbiturates
          b. Abuse: narcotics, alcohol
          c. Reaction: anaphylaxis
     (ii) Plants, chemicals, heavy metals
     (iiii) Stings, bites
3. Endogenous causes
     (i) Glucose: hypoglycaemia, diabetic ketoacidosis
     (ii) Acid-base disturbances
     (iii) Electrolyte disturbances, hyper/hyponatraemia, hyper-
           /hypokalaemia
     (iv) Organ failure: renal, hepatic, adrenal
     (v) Burns encephalopathy
     (vi) Inborn errors of amino acids, organic acids, urea cycle etc
4. Shock e.g. asphyxia, septicaemia, trauma, heart failure etc
5. Hypertensive encephalopathy (p. 102)
6. Hysteria

CAUSES OF RAISED INTRACRANIAL PRESSURE

1. Hydrocephalus
2. Intracranial bleed
     (i) Neonatal: intraventricular haemorrhage, rupture of vessels,
          venous sinuses, thalamic bleeds
     (ii) Trauma: subdural
     (iii) Arterio-venous malformation
     (iv) Dural sinus thrombosis

3. Traumatic brain swelling
4. Infection: meningitis, encephalitis
5. Mass lesion, abscess, leukaemia, tumour
6. Toxic encephalopathy, e.g. Reye's syndrome
7. Benign intracranial hypertension

CAUSES OF NYSTAGMUS

1. Ocular — pendular nystagmus
   (i) Astigmatism
   (ii) Cataracts, retrolental fibroplasia
   (iii) Congenital
   (iv) Albinism
2. Vestibular — varies with head position
   (i) Labyrinthine
      a. Infection, e.g. mumps, encephalitis
      b. Benign paroxysmal vertigo
      c. Ménières disease (rare)
   (ii) Vestibular
      a. Neuronitis, e.g. otitis media
      b. Gentamycin
3. Cerebellar and brain stem — increased on looking laterally
   (i) Infection, e.g. encephalitis, TB meningitis
   (ii) Drugs, e.g. phenytoin, barbiturates
   (iii) Injury, e.g. hydrocephalus, cerebral palsy, trauma
   (iv) Tumour: cerebellar astrocytoma, medulloblastoma,
        neuroblastoma
   (v) Degenerations, e.g. Friedreich's ataxia, ataxia-telangiectasia
        (p. 82) etc
4. Environmental — intermittent nystagmus: Spasmus nutans

Causes of acute cerebellar ataxia
1. Infection
   (i) Viral: chickenpox, polio, Echo, infectious mononucleosis,
       coxsackie, measles, rubella
   (ii) Bacterial: meningitis, cerebellar abscess
2. Drugs e.g. piperazine, phenytoin, alcohol, DDT
3. Trauma, anoxia
4. Raised intracranial pressure
5. Seizure
6. Hysteria
7. Migraine
8. Hypoglycaemia

Causes of chronic cerebellar ataxia
1. Hydrocephalus
2. Cerebral palsy

3. Tumour:
   (i) posterior fossa cerebellar astrocytoma, medulloblastoma
   (ii) extracranial occult neuroblastoma
4. Metabolic, e.g. lead, hypothyroidism, Hartnup's disease, arginino-succinic aciduria abetalipoproteinaemia, maple syrup urine disease
5. Degenerations, e.g. ataxia telangiectasia, Friedreich's ataxia, storage diseases (p. 153), multiple sclerosis, etc

CAUSES OF HYPOTONIA OR FLOPPY INFANT

1. Non-paralytic (hypotonia without significant weakness)
   (i) Non-neurological
       a. Acute infection
       b. Failure to thrive, malabsorption
       c. Prematurity, any severe neonatal disease
       d. Ligamentous laxity
       e. Metabolic: scurvy, rickets, hypothyroidism, renal tubular acidosis, hypercalcaemia
   (ii) Neurological
       a. Mental retardation
       b. Birth asphyxia, injury
       c. Down's syndrome
       d. Cerebral palsy
       e. Metabolic: amino acidurias, storage disorders (p. 153)
       f. Prader-Willi, Riley-Day syndromes
2. Paralytic (weakness with incidental hypotonia)
   (i) Spinal cord
       a. Trauma e.g. birth injury
       b. Poliomyelitis
       c. Spinal muscular atrophy, early (Werdnig-Hoffman) and late
   (ii) Peripheral nerve
       a. Polyneuritis e.g. Guillaine-Barré, hypertrophic interstitial polyneuritis (rare)
       b. Heavy metal poisoning: lead, cadmium
   (iii) Neuromuscular junction: myasthenia gravis
   (iv) Myopathic disorders
       a. Progressive e.g. Duchênne muscular dystrophy, Pompe's disease (p. 152)
       b. Non-progressive e.g. central core, nemaline rod disease, myotonia congenita
       c. Polymyositis
       d. Metabolic e.g. steroids, thyroid dysfunction, periodic paralyses of McArdle's syndrome, hypohyperkalaemia etc
   (v) Unknown: benign congenital hypotonia

CAUSES OF CRANIOTABES (skull so thin as to allow it to be indented like a ping-pong ball)

1. Physiological to 3 months
2. Hydrocephalus
3. Rickets
4. Rare: syphilis, osteogenesis imperfecta, hypervitaminosis A

CAUSES OF DELAYED CLOSURE OF ANTERIOR FONTANELLE (normally by 2 years)

1. Metabolic
   - (i) Rickets, malnutrition
   - (ii) Hypothyroidism
   - (iii) Mucopolysaccharidoses
   - (iv) Hypophosphatasia
2. Hydrocephalus
3. Infection: congenital rubella, syphilis
4. Chromosome trisomies: Down's, 17–18, 13–15
5. Rare: achondroplasia, cleido-cranial dysostosis, Russell-Silver dwarf, progeria

CAUSES OF A SMALL HEAD

1. Normal CNS
   - (i) Normal variation
   - (ii) Familial
   - (iii) Small, in proportion to body
2. Abnormal CNS likely, disproportionately small
   - (i) Microcephaly: familial, sporadic, post brain injury, part of mental retardation syndrome

CAUSES OF A LARGE HEAD

1. Normal central nervous system
   - (i) Normal variation
   - (ii) Familial
   - (iii) Marked disproportion of body: premature, failure to thrive
   - (iv) Haemoglobinopathies: sickle cell, thalassaemia major
2. Abnormal central nervous system likely
   - (i) Hydrocephalus
   - (ii) Space occupying lesion
   - (iii) Megalencephaly: degenerative disorders, neurofibromatosis, idiopathic, achondroplasia, mucopolysaccharidosis
   - (iv) Craniostenosis of sagittal suture
   - (v) Sotos syndrome

CAUSES OF SOME UNUSUAL SKULL X-RAY APPEARANCES

1. Copper beating
   (i) Hydrocephalus — spina bifida complex
   (ii) Physiological
2. Calcification
   (i) Physiological: choroid, falx, clinoid ligaments
   (ii) Neurodermatoses: Sturge-Weber syndrome, tuberous sclerosis
   (iii) Trauma, haemorrhage
   (iv) Inflammation
       a. Congenital toxoplasmosis, cytomegalovirus
       b. Pyogenic abscess, tuberculosis
       c. Cystercicosis, echinococcus
   (v) Neoplastic: craniopharyngioma, dermoid, teratoma, astrocytoma etc
   (vi) Metabolic: hyper-/hypoparathyroidism, vitamin D excess

CAUSES OF CATARACTS

1. Unknown
2. Congenital: rubella, familial
3. Early onset: galactosaemia, low birth weight, Lowe's oculo-cerebro-renal dystrophy, Hurler's, Gm_1 gangliosidosis (p. 154)
4. Late onset: Down's syndrome, myotonic dystrophy, diabetes mellitus

CAUSES OF A WHITE PUPILLARY REFLEX

1. Cataract
2. Retinoblastoma
3. Congenital: coloboma, choroidoretinitis, etc
4. Retinal detachment, e.g. non-accidental injury
5. Retrolental fibroplasia
6. Intra-ocular foreign body
7. Toxocara canis

FURTHER READING

Brett E M 1983 Paediatric neurology. Churchill Livingstone, Edinburgh
Hall D B M 1984 The child with a handicap. Blackwell Scientific, Oxford
Robinson R 1984 When to start and stop anticonvulsants. In: Meadow R (ed) Recent advances in paediatrics 7. Churchill Livingstone, Edinburgh, pp. 155–174.
Stone F H, Koupernik C 1985 Child psychiatry for students. 3rd edn. Churchill Livingstone, Edinburgh

Behaviour

NORMAL SEQUENCE OF RESPONSES TO MAJOR STRESSFUL EVENT

Seen in older children and parents to chronic illness, e.g. diabetes, and bereavement
1. Shock, recognition and, often, denial
2. Anger
3. Guilt
4. Acceptance, allowing constructive action

Each stage may last months or years and merge into each other. Complete restitution may not occur

COMMON BEHAVIOURS WHICH IN EXCESS OR PROLONGED DURATION ARE ABNORMAL

1. Repetitive actions e.g. head banging or rolling, body rocking: consider emotional disturbance, mental retardation
2. Pica: consider anaemia, lead posioning
3. Masturbation: consider emotional disturbance

CAUSES OF ENURESIS

1. Physiological delay (with family history usual)
2. Psychological stress
3. Organic
    (i) Urinary tract infection
    (ii) Mental retardation
    (iii) Neurological e.g. spina bifida, epilepsy
    (iv) Structural lesion e.g. posterior urethral valves
    (v) Diabetes mellitus

CAUSES OF FAECAL SOILING

1. Untrained
2. Organic: anal fissure resulting in constipation and overflow incontinence, Hirschsprung's disease

3. Psychological
    (i) Retention, may lead to fissure!
    (ii) Antisocial

CAUSES OF RECURRENT ABDOMINAL PAIN/PERIODIC SYNDROME

1. Psychological stress
    (i) Home: marital discord, separation experiences, family illness, poor parent–child relationship
    (ii) School: bullying, problems in discipline and learning
    (iii) Sexual abuse
2. Migraine tendency: personal and family history
3. Constipation
4. Medical causes of acute and recurrent abdominal pain (pp. 113, 115)

CAUSES OF SCHOOL REFUSAL

1. School phobia: separation anxiety, refuses to leave
2. Truancy: leaves home and fails to arrive or absconds later. Educational difficulties, psychosocial problems common
3. Educational difficulties e.g. slow, chronic illness, poor vision, unsuspected hearing loss, emotional stress, dyslexia etc, poor teaching, large class

CAUSES OF REPETITIVE MOVEMENTS OR TICS

1. Tics: stress, unknown causes
2. Stammer: purposeless 'displacement' movements common in older child with severe stutter
3. Drugs: phenothiazines, haloperidol, metoclopramide, imipramine
4. Hyperthyroidism (other signs usually present)
5. Chorea: (see rheumatic fever p. 103) cerebral palsy, Sydenham's, Wilson's disease, Huntington's

CAUSES OF CHRONIC LASSITUDE

1. Emotional
    (i) Depression
    (ii) School refusal
    (iii) Grief
2. Lack of sleep
3. Infections: glandular fever, tuberculosis, chronic infections
4. Anaemia
5. Malignancy
6. Endocrine: thyroid and adrenal cortex disease
7. Others: cardiac, renal, rheumatoid, myasthenia etc

Respiratory disease

EXAMINATION OF THE NOSE

Check shape, deviation and nasal discharge (unilateral, mucopurulent/bloody in foreign body or choanal atresia). A transverse crease suggests allergy from frequent rubbing of the nose with the flat of the hand (allergic salute).

The mucosa can be seen with the auriscope light, and in older children the speculum can be used to assess it. Pink is normal, red infected, pale and swollen allergic/vasomotor rhinitis, and Little's area often has scars or ulcers from nose picking and associated bleeds. Polyps occur in older children with cystic fibrosis. Mouth breathing in mid-childhood suggests adenoidal hypertrophy. Tonsils and adenoids largest at 6–8 years

EXAMINATION OF THE EARS

Note shape, position (below a line level with the outer canthus of the eye suggests renal abnormality) and size.

To examine the tympanic membrane in the younger child demonstrate examination on a doll/parent and invite imitation, then jointly handling the auriscope with the child or you alone examine the child's ear.

If potentially uncooperative the infant or child is sat facing forwards or sideways on an adult's lap, head held against the adult's chest with one hand, the other hand round the child's hands and trunk.

To straighten the external auditory canal for the best view
infant: pull the ear lobe downwards
child: pull pinna (top) up and back
To prevent injury or pain from a sudden movement of the child rest the knuckles of the hand holding the auriscope on the cheek or scalp

Causes of changes in appearance of the tympanic membrane (TM)
Grey drum, with cone of light reflex, is normal
1. Pink injection around the edge of the TM in crying infant
2. Red uniformly in acute otitis media

3. Dark, almost black in impending perforation or blood behind TM
4. Black hole is a perforation
5. Dull grey retracted TM in blocked eustachian tube
6. Dull grey bulging TM, often with bubbles or a fluid level, in secretory otitis

EXAMINATION OF THE CHEST

Respiratory rate: infancy   40 ± 10 per minute
                 child   30 ± 10 per minute
                 adult   15 ± 5 per minute

A. Observation
Rounded diameter in infancy, oval thereafter.

Costochondral junctions seen or palpated along a line from mid-clavicle obliquely down to the anterior axillary line at the bottom of the rib cage. The junctions are enlarged in rickets (rickety rosary).

Harrison's sulci are the depressions along the lower rib cage at the insertion of diaphragmatic muscle, normal or due to chronic respiratory or cardiac disease, or rickets.

As the front of the chest is of soft cartilage the sternum is indrawn in generalised lung collapse, e.g. respiratory distress syndrome, or airways obstruction, e.g. epiglottitis; hyperinflation in bronchiolitis or asthma produces a pigeon chest appearance

B. Percussion
Infants: chest wall and contents hyper-resonant, increased if lying on a mattress, which acts as a sounding board, and percussion not very helpful. Can identify the upper boarder of the liver on the right (6th space anteriorly, decreasing dullness up to the 4th space).
Children: findings in pneumonia, effusions, and hyperinflation similar to adults

C. Auscultation
Breath sounds are bronchial in infancy, and remain so over the mid-clavicular areas in small children. Similar sound heard in consolidation, lobar collapse.

Upper respiratory noises may be referred and often cause confusion but are coarse crackles, not medium or fine crackles due to bronchitis/bronchopneumonia.

Fine crackles are heard in pneumonia, and expiratory wheeze, with fine crackles in infants with bronchiolitis and medium crackles in asthma

SIGNS OF ACUTE RESPIRATORY DISTRESS
1. Restlessness, agitation
2. Cyanosis

3. Stridor
    (i) Inspiratory, progressing sometimes to inspiratory and
        expiratory in supraglottic or glottic obstruction
    (ii) Expiratory stridor more prominent in subglottic obstruction
4. Flaring of alae naesi
5. Head retraction with neck extension
6. Marked sternal retraction in obstructed airways or lung collapse
    e.g. epiglottitis, respiratory distress syndrome
7. Hyperinflation of chest in air trapping e.g. bronchiolitis, asthma

SOME DEFINITIONS

Atopy: Altered reactivity to allergens, genetically predisposed,
causing hay fever, eczema and asthma

Bronchiolitis: Respiratory syncitial virus related to acute
inflammation of bronchioles causing wheeze in infants less than
6 months old. No increased personal or family history of atopy.
About half have repeated wheeze (wheezy baby syndrome)

Wheezy baby syndrome: Repeated wheeze generally
unresponsive to bronchodilators or steroids, following viral
infections in infants aged 6 to 12 months. Steady regression of
symptoms in early childhood; the majority do not have atopy or
go on to develop asthma

Asthma: Episodic airway obstruction reversed by
bronchodilators and/or steroids. Onset from 1 to 5 years of age in
individuals with a personal or family history of atopy, and
precipitated by viral infections

FORCED EXPIRATION TESTS OF LUNG FUNCTION

(The most commonly used tests clinically, the norms are related to
the height of children, not their age). Results are tabulated as the
best of 3 attempts

1. Peak expiratory flow rate (PEFR). The highest flow achieved in
    the first tenth of a second of expiration measured with a Wright
    peak flow meter. Although effort dependent it is very
    reproducible in children over 3 years old, and is the most
    commonly used test to monitor progress and therapy in
    asthmatics at home as well as in hospital
2. Forced vital capacity (FVC). The total volume of gas expelled
    during forced expiration. Drawbacks include limitation to the
    over-5s, and being dependent on the children's effort. FVC is
    reduced in small lungs, stiff lungs, scoliosis or neuromuscular
    disease
3. Forced expiratory volume (FEV). The volume of gas expired in
    the first second is the FEV_1. It is disproportionately reduced to
    below 80% of the FVC in airway obstruction, e.g. asthma, cystic
    fibrosis

4. Exercise test of bronchial responsiveness used in diagnosis of asthma and assessment of treatment. The standardised test is exercise on a treadmill or bicycle ergometer for 6–8 minutes with heart rate at least 170 beats per minute. A positive response is a fall of 15% or more from baseline in PEFR or FEV_1 taken at 0, 5, 10, 15, 20 and 25 minutes from the end of exercise. Peak broncho-constriction is usually at 3–7 minutes

Relation of age to infectious respiratory illness

Age	*Illness*	*Bacteria*	*Viruses*
Neonatal	Pneumonia	E. coli Pseudomonas Group B haem. strep	Respiratory syncitial virus (RSV)
Infancy	Bronchiolitis Wheezy baby syndrome	— —	RSV Parainfluenza Adenovirus Rhinovirus
	Broncho-pneumonia	Staph. aureus Strep. pneumoniae	RSV Parainfluenza Adenovirus Rhinovirus Influenza Measles
Toddler (1–3 years)	Laryngo-tracheitis Broncho-pneumonia	Strep. pneumoniae	As in infancy
	Asthma	Mycoplasma pneumonia (uncommon)	Rhinovirus RSV Parainfluenza etc
3–7 years	Epiglottitis	Haemophilus influenzae	Parainfluenza Influenza Adenovirus RVS
School age (4+ years)	Broncho-pneumonia	Strep. pneumoniae Mycoplasma pneumoniae	Adenovirus Parainfluenza Influenza Cytomegalovirus Measles
All ages	Recurrent otitis media, upper respiratory tract infection	Strep. pneumoniae H. influenzae	RSV Adenovirus Influenza Parainfluenza

CAUSES OF ACUTE COUGH

1. Acute respiratory infections
    (i) Upper: colds, tonsillitis, pharyngitis
    (ii) Laryngeal: laryngitis, epiglottitis
    (iii) Lower: bronchiolitis, bronchitis, pneumonia
2. Asthma, wheezy bronchitis
3. Pertussis, pertussis syndrome e.g. adenovirus, parainfluenza
4. Foreign body

CAUSES OF CHRONIC COUGH

1. Postnasal drip: colds, atopic adenoids, sinusitis
2. Asthma
3. Infection
    (i) Viruses causing tracheitis, bronchitis, partial lung collapse
    (ii) Tuberculosis
    (iii) Mycoplasma, psittacosis
4. Post-pertussis
5. Foreign body
6. Cystic fibrosis
7. Recurrent aspiration: hiatus hernia, achalasia, tracheo-oesophageal fistula
8. Extrinsic compression of trachea or bronchus e.g. glands, tumour, heart enlargement
9. Habit
10. Rare: extrinsic allergic alveolitis, pulmonary haemosiderosis

DIFFERENTIATION OF THE MAJOR CAUSES OF ACUTE STRIDOR, epiglottitis (E), laryngotracheobronchitis (LTB) and foreign body (FB) above the carina

	E	LTB	FB
Age	0–3 years	3–7 years	≥6 months
Onset	In hours	1–2 days	Sudden, may be missed
Respirations	Laboured	Increased	Variable
Cough	+	++	+++
Drooling	+++	−	−
Appearance	Pale, toxic	Normal/anxious	Normal
Voice	Hoarse, weak	Hoarse	May be aphonic
Hypoxia	Frequent	Unusual	Variable
X-ray:			
neck	Large epiglottis	Normal	Radio- opaque FB?
chest	Normal	Inflammatory changes in half the children	Lung or lobe overinflated/collapsed if FB moves below carina

CAUSES OF ACUTE STRIDOR

1. Acute laryngotracheobronchitis
2. Acute epiglottitis
3. Foreign body
4. Measles, glandular fever
5. Rare but important: diphtheria, retropharyngeal abscess, acute angioneurotic oedema

CAUSES OF CHRONIC STRIDOR

1. Weak cartilage in the wall: laryngomalacia
2. Internal narrowing
   (i) Subglottic stenosis or haemangioma
   (ii) Vocal cord paralysis: recurrent laryngeal nerve damage, raised intracranial pressure
   (iii) Laryngeal web, papilloma
3. Obstruction
   (i) Tongue in micrognathia (Pierre-Robin syndrome)
   (ii) Tonsils and adenoids in sleep apnoea/Pickwickian syndrome of somnolence, cyanosis, cor pulmonale +/− obesity
4. Compression from surrounding structures: vascular ring, tumour, cystic hygroma, retrosternal goitre

CAUSES OF GENERALISED LYMPHADENOPATHY

1. Infection
   (i) Bacterial: TB, typhoid, brucellosis, pyogenic
   (ii) Viral: rubella, measles, glandular fever, cytomegalovirus, Aids-related complex, cat scratch fever
   (iii) Other: toxoplasmosis, syphilis, malaria
2. Eczema
3. Collagenoses e.g. Still's disease
4. Medication: phenytoin, serum sickness
5. Malignancies: leukaemia, lymphoma, histiocytosis X
6. Chronic granulomatous disease
7. Storage disease: Gaucher's, Niemann-Pick's

CAUSES OF LOCALISED LYMPHADENOPATHY

1. Infection — see above
2. Metastases — see above
3. Immunisation e.g. BCG in arm
4. Lymphoma
5. Kawasaki disease: cervical

CAUSES OF PNEUMONIA

1. Infection
   (i) Viral in 90%
   (ii) Bacterial   (see p. 79 for organisms)
2. Aspiration syndromes
   (i) Prematurity
   (ii) Hiatus hernia, tracheo-oesophageal fistula, chalasia of oesophagus
   (iii) Drugs, epilepsy, anaesthesia
   (iv) Kerosene, paraffin, zinc stearate (baby powder)
3. Foreign body
4. Cystic fibrosis: staphylococcus aureus, pseudomonas
5. Immunological incompetence, primary or secondary: common organisms, Candida, aspergillus, pneumocystis carinii
6. Extrinsic allergic alveolitis
7. Loeffler syndrome: ascaris, toxocara canis
8. Miscellaneous: paraquat, collagenoses

TRIGGERS CAUSING ASTHMA ATTACKS

1. Extrinsic
   (i) Inhaled: housedust mite, animal hair, feathers, mould spores, pollens
   (ii) Oral: tartrazine, cola drinks, ice, milk, chocolate
2. Infection: rhinovirus, parainfluenza, respiratory syncitial virus
3. Exercise
4. Emotion
5. Weather changes, cold air, moist air
6. Chemicals: paint and kerosene fumes
7. Aspirin sensitivity (rare)

CAUSES OF RECURRENT WHEEZE

1. Reactive airways: asthma, bronchioloitis, wheezy baby syndrome, extrinsic allergic alveolitis
2. Mechanical: foreign body, compression from mediastinal glands, tumours, aberrant vessels
3. Infections: post-pertussis, Löffler's syndrome
4. Mendelian genetic disease: cystic fibrosis, immotile cilia syndrome, including Kartegener syndrome, α_1 antitrypsin deficiency, immunodeficiencies
5. Aspiration syndromes (p. 82)
6. Congestive cardiac failure
7. Congenital lung abnormality: bronchogenic cyst, sequestrated lobe, lobar emphysema, cystic adenomatous malformation

CAUSES OF ACUTE RESPIRATORY FAILURE

1. Bronchopneumonia
2. Accidents: trauma, burns, drowning, poisoning, foreign body
3. Upper airway obstruction (see causes of stridor, p. 81)
4. Septicaemia
5. Encephalitis, seizures
6. Congenital heart disease
7. Status asthmaticus
8. Intrathoracic anomalies: diaphragmatic lesion, vascular ring, lobar emphysema
9. Peripheral neuritis

CAUSES OF SEGMENTAL COLLAPSE (ATELECTASIS)

A. Neonatal
1. Parenchymal
    (i) Respiratory distress syndrome
    (ii) Pneumonia
    (iii) Meconium aspiration
2. Displacement
    (i) Intrathoracic: pneumothorax, lobar emphysema, tumour
    (ii) Extrathoracic: ascites

B. Infancy up to 1 year old
1. Parenchymal
    (i) Pneumonia, recurrent aspiration syndromes (p. 82) immune-deficiencies, immotile cilia
    (ii) Pertussis
    (iii) Bronchopulmonary dysplasia
    (iv) Cystic fibrosis
    (v) Bronchiolitis obliterans (post-adenovirus)
2. Intraluminal
    (i) Bronchiolitis
    (ii) Intubation, post-extubation
    (iii) Stenosis of trachea or bronchus, hypoplastic airways
3. Extraluminal
    (i) Hilar glands, cysts, tumours
    (ii) Aberrant vessels, vascular ring
    (iii) Congenital heart disease with enlarged left atrium

C. Child
1. Parenchymal
    (i) Pneumonia
    (ii) Cystic fibrosis, bronchiectasis
    (iii) Tuberculosis
    (iv) Post-operative
    (v) Neuromuscular weakness, immobility

2. Intraluminal
   (i) Asthma
   (ii) Foreign body
   (iii) As in B.2.(ii) and (iii) above
3. Extraluminal, as in B.3.(i)–(iii) above

X-RAY DIFFERENCES BETWEEN CONSOLIDATION AND COLLAPSE (ATELECTASIS)

	Consolidation	Collapse
Mediastinal shift	–	+ towards lesion
Compensatory hyperinflation of other lobes	–	+
Fissure position	unchanged	+ towards lesion
Diaphragm on same side	Unchanged	elevated
Air bronchogram	+	variable

CAUSES OF PERSISTENT OR RECURRENT LUNG FIELD INFILTRATES ON X-RAY

1. Infections
   (i) Partially treated bacterial infections
   (ii) TB, mycoplasma, psittacosis, pertussis, cytomegalovirus, Löffler's syndrome, pneumocystis carinii
2. Asthma
3. Aspiration syndromes (see causes of pneumonia, p. 82)
4. Foreign body
5. Left to right cardiac shunt
6. Cystic fibrosis
7. Malignancy: leukaemia, histiocytosis, lymphomas
8. Drugs: nitrofurantoin, methotrexate
9. Neonatal
   (i) Bronchopulmonary dysplasia, Wilson-Mikity pulmonary dysmaturity syndrome in prematures
   (ii) Congenital rubella, cytomegalovirus, syphilis

CAUSES OF BILATERAL HYPERINFLATION

1. Asthma
2. Bronchiolitis
3. Acute laryngo-tracheo-bronchitis
4. Cystic fibrosis
5. Interstitial pneumonitis

CAUSES OF UNILATERAL LUNG HYPERTRANSLUCENCY ON X-RAY

1. Compensatory hyperinflation, opposite side pneumonia, aspiration
2. Pneumothorax
3. Lobar emphysema
   (i) Foreign body
   (ii) Bronchial compression   } 'ball valve' effect
   (iii) Congenital
4. Pulmonary and bronchogenic cysts, pneumatocoeles
5. Bronchiolitis obliterans
6. Unknown

CAUSES OF UNILATERAL OPACIFICATION ON X-RAY

1. Pneumonia
2. Tension pneumothorax of opposite lung
3. Aspiration
4. Haemothorax
5. Pleural effusion: tuberulosis, infective, malignancy
6. Empyema
7. Diaphragmatic hernia
8. Chylothorax
9. Agenesis of the lung

DIFFERENTIAL DIAGNOSIS OF MEDIASTINAL MASSES

Anterior
1. Lymphoreticular system
   (i) Normal thymus
   (ii) Thymic tumour
   (iii) Lymph nodes
2. Goitre
3. Congenital: dermoid, cystic hygroma

Middle
1. Lymph nodes: TB, leukaemia, lymphoma
2. Bronchogenic cyst
3. Pericardial cyst

Posterior
1. Gastrointestinal tract:
   (i) oesophagus: hiatal hernia, achalasia
   (ii) reduplication, neurenteric cyst
2. Neurogenic tumour: ganglioneuroma, neuroblastoma
3. Paravertebral abscess
4. Anterior meningocoele

X-RAY APPEARANCES OF NOTE

Common normal X-ray appearances (Fig. 7)

1. Ossification centre, upper sternum. Coin-like, it may be confusing if the child is slightly rotated and it is then seen in the lung field
2. Sail sign of a normal thymus
3. Slightly increased bronchovascular markings in the right lower zone *only*, no thickening or segmental opacities in health
4. Wave sign of normal thymus indented by overlying intercostal muscles
5. Fat line extends beyond lung fields, and lung markings extend to the periphery unlike in pneumothorax

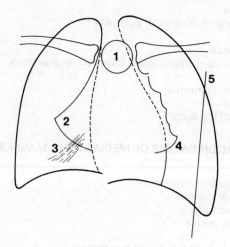

Fig. 7

X-ray signs of pneumonia in sites often overlooked (Fig. 8)

1. Right upper lobe, upper segment
2. Middle lobe, medial segment. Not to be confused with normal bronchovascular markings
3. Left lower lobe i.e. always look *behind* the heart shadow
4. Small effusion at the costophrenic angle

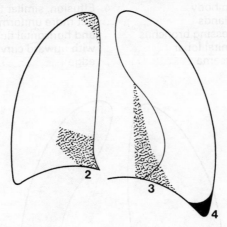

Fig. 8

X-ray appearance in asthma/bronchiolitis (Fig. 9)

Features to identify:
   barrel chest shape
   horizontal ribs
   flat diaphragms
   prominent hilar bronchovascular markings
   hypertranslucent lung fields

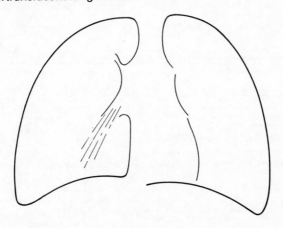

Fig. 9

Common causes of asymmetric lungfield translucency on X-ray
(Fig. 10)

1. Compensatory hyperinflation for collapse of other lung
2. Pneumothorax
3. Ball-valve effect
   (i) Foreign body
   (ii) Hilar glands compressing bronchus
   (iii) Congenital lobar emphysema

1. Pneumonia
2. Tension pneumothorax *other* lung, this one collapsed
3. Aspiration into lung
4. Effusion, similar to aspiration but more uniform opacity and horizontal fluid level with upward curve at lung edge

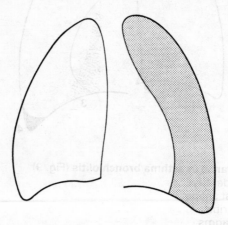

Fig. 10

X-ray appearances in cystic fibrosis (Fig. 11)

Early signs:
  hyperinflation
  segmental/lobar collapse
  especially right upper
  and middle lobes

Later signs:
cystic areas, thickened bronchial
walls, well seen end on. Left
upper and right middle
particularly affected.
Scars show as thickened lines
radiating from the hilum

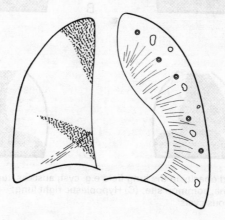

Fig. 11

X-ray appearances in staphylococcal pneumonia (Fig. 12)

1. Pneumothorax
2. Effusion (empyema) } pyopneumothorax
3. Cysts, often fluid fille

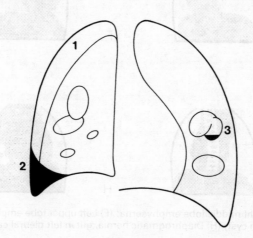

Fig. 12

SOME CHEST X-RAY ABNORMALITIES IN INFANCY

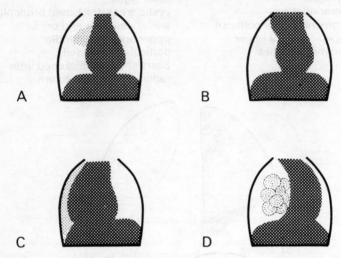

Fig. 13 (A) Round opacity in the lung field e.g. cyst, abscess, tumour;
(B) Neuroblastoma, common site; (C) Hypoplastic right lung;
(D) Emphysematous cysts

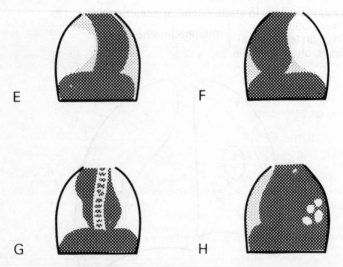

Fig. 14 (E) Right middle lobe emphyserna; (F) Left upper lobe emphysena;
(G) Duplication cyst; (H) Diaphrogmatic hernia, gut in left pleural cavity

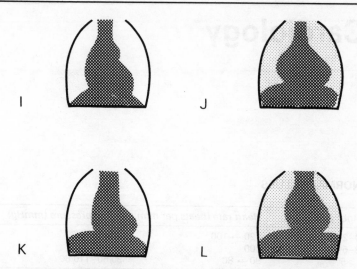

Fig. 15 (I) Post-stenotic dilatation of pulmonary artery; (J) Transposition of the great arteries; (K) Fallot's tetralogy 'boot shaped heart'; (L) Pulmonary plethora: (i) acyanotic L → R shunt of VSD, PDA, ASD (ii) cyanotic TGA

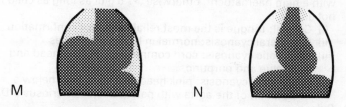

Fig. 16 (M) Eventration of diaphragm; (N) Total anomalous pulmonary venous drainage 'cottage loaf'

RECOMMENDED READING

Phelan P, Landau L, Olinsky A 1982 Respiratory illness in childhood. Blackwell, Oxford

Silverman M 1985 Asthma in childhood. Current Medical Literature Ltd, London

Cardiology

NORMAL VALUES

Age (years)	Heart rate (beats per min)	Blood pressure (mmHg)
0–2	120 → 100	80/50–90/60
3–5	100	90/60
>5	90 → 80	90/60–110/80

EXAMINATION

1. Cyanosis = >5 g/dl of desaturated Haemoglobin(Hb) in newborn with a high haematocrit, otherwise >1.5 g/dl as long as child is not anaemic
   - (i) Central: tongue is the most reliable site for confirmation
   - (ii) Peripheral cyanosis: normal in healthy neonates
   - (iii) Traumatic cyanosis: cord compression makes head and neck blue and purpuric
   - (iv) Differential cyanosis: pink head and neck, blue below a coarctation of the aorta with patent ductus arteriosus (PDA)

2. Pulse
   Always check femoral pulses.
   Absence, weakness or delay compared with right radial or axilla pulse suggests coarctation. Check blood pressure (BP): see 3. below; lower BP in legs confirms coarctation

3. Blood pressure (BP)
   Cuff size two-thirds the length of the outer aspect of the upper arm or thigh, ensuring its bladder encircles the limb.
   BP in legs normally 20 mm Hg higher than arms
   Procedure in infants: Auscultation often difficult in babies, so flush BP may be used. Raise the limb, apply cuff, inflate, lower the limb — a red blush as the cuff is slowly deflated approximates to the mean systolic BP. Doppler is now replacing this time honoured method
   Procedure in children: Toddlers and children respond well to making a game of it. 'Let's play the silver line game. You look for it (the mercury column), and I'll listen.' Inflate, check radial or

dorsalis pedis pulse as you deflate to get idea of systolic (may be the only reading!). Palpate for brachial or popliteal pulsation, apply stethoscope to the spot, and repeat. Diastolic may be indeterminate in otherwise healthy children, i.e. does not disappear until down to 20–30 mm Hg

4. Apex
   4th or 5th interspace, within the nipple line
   Always check for dextrocardia
5. Liver edge
   Easily palpated in infants and toddlers (p. 107), 1–3 cm below the right costal margin in the nipple line
6. Jugular venous pressure
   Useful in older children. Hepatomegaly is a more reliable sign of congestive cardiac failure in the 0–2 year old
7. Oedema
   Infants and sick children lie horizontally, so look for pitting oedema over the sacrum, or swelling around eyes
8. Surgical scars tell their own story
   Cut down sites for drips, femoral scars of catheters. Sterniotomy scar from cardiac surgery. Thoracotomy scar for PDA, to make shunts for cyanotic congenital heart problems, lung or mediastinal problems. Neck and upper abdomen scars for lines and CSF shunts.

Auscultation
In addition to the 4 major sites, listen over the second left anterior intercostal space (patent ductus murmur best heart here) and the (upper for ductus, lower for VSD).
   Auscultate in both supine and sitting positions
1. Serious heart disease *does* occur without a murmur. Myocarditis is then more likely than congenital lesion
2. Rapid heart rate may obscure abnormal heart sounds and murmurs
3. Venous hums are often continuous and subclavicular. If heard on the left may be confused with a PDA. Turning the head or lying down alters a hum but not a ductus murmur
4. Innocent murmurs
   (i) Asymptomatic
   (ii) No thrill
   (iii) Localised to the left sternal border and apex
   (iv) Short and musical, mid-systolic and grade 3/6 or less
   (v) Varies with sitting up and lying down, often disappears on lying
5. Third heart sound is physiological, in early diastole, at the apex, best heard in left lateral position

IMPORTANT PATHOLOGICAL FINDINGS

First sound
An ejection click follows immediately after it in post stenotic
dilatation of the pulmonary artery or aorta and due to rapid filling

Second sound
Loud in pulmonary hypertension.
Soft and apparently single in isolated pulmonary stenosis and
Fallot's tetralogy.
Fixed split on breathing in/out in atrial septal defect

Murmurs

Ejection systolic
Increased flow or stenosis of pulmonary or aortic valve

Pansystolic
1. Shunt from higher to lower pressure e.g. ventricular septal
   defect (VSD), primum type atrial septal defect (ASD), patent
   ductus arteriosus (PDA)
2. Regurgitant e.g. mitral incompetence

Diastolic
(diaphragm)	early	=	regurgitant aorta or pulmonary valve
(bell)	middle	=	increased flow from shunts (VSD, ASD, PDA)
(bell)	late	=	obstructed flow across 'tight' tricuspid or mitral valve

Continuous
1. Patent ductus arteriosus (unusual in infancy)
2. Combinations of AS and AI, MI and AI, VSD and AI
3. Coarctation of the aorta (due to collaterals, best heard over the
   back, in child over 5 years old)

CONGENITAL HEART DISEASE

Frequency of congenital heart defects is 6 per 1000 children.
Relative frequency: VSD = 30%, PDA = 15%, other < 10% each

Acyanotic congenital heart disease — shunts*

	Age specific symptoms	Clinical signs of note
Patent ductus arteriosus	Premature: recurrent apnoea, persistent RDS, CCF Infant: 'chesty', FTT, CCF Adult: breathless, cyanosis, SBE	Pulses: bounding Thrill: 'to and fro' left infraclavicular area, same as Murmurs: pansystolic, becoming continuous and 'machinery' like ± mid-diastolic flow murmur from mitral valve at apex
Ventricular septal defect	3 months: large VSD — reduced pulmonary vascular resistance causes acute CCF ± cyanosis Infant: moderate VSD — 'chesty', FTT, CCF Child: small VSD — asymptomatic, risk of SBE	Pulse: normal, or weak and rapid Apex: thrusting, laterally displaced Thrill: lower left sternal edge Heart sounds: second is widely split, from increased filling of right ventricle Murmurs: harsh pansystolic ± mid-diastolic mitral flow at apex
Atrial septal defect:		
Ostium secundum	Child: asymptomatic Adult: breathless from pulmonary hypertension	Pulse: normal, no thrill Heart sounds: wide fixed split of second sound from conduction delay (right bundle branch block) Murmurs: mid-systolic at 2nd left interspace, ± mid-diastolic tricuspid flow at lower right sternal edge
Ostium primum	Infant: 'chesty', FTT, CCF Child: progressive cyanosis as shunt reverses from the pulmonary hypertension	As for secundum, + if mitral valve is cleft (common): Thrill: left sternal edge Murmur: apical pansystolic from mitral valve incompetence

* N. B. Chest X-ray in all but the mildest cases shows varying degrees of cardiac enlargement, pulmonary plethora and prominent pulmonary vessels

CCF = Congestive cardiac failure; FTT = failure to thrive; RDS = Respiratory distress syndrome; SBE = subacute bacterial endocarditis; VSD = ventricular septal defect

Acyanotic congenital heart disease — obstructive

	Age specific symptoms	Clinical signs of note
Aortic stenosis (various causes)	Infancy: (i) valvular — CCF if a severe stenosis; (ii) supravalvular — asymptomatic, unusual face, retarded development. ↑ Ca++ (William's syndrome) Child & adult: valve/obstructive cardiomyopathy — dizzy, angina, sudden death	Pulse: small volume, 'plateau' Apex: thrust Thrill: left sternal edge radiating up to the neck Heart sounds: soft 2nd aortic part, the usual split may be reversed (i.e. ↑ on expiration) Murmur: ejection systolic radiating to the neck
Coarctation of the aorta	Infancy: breathless, CCF (VSD often present) Child & adult: asymptomatic, rarely ruptured berry aneurysm, SBE	Differential cyanosis in neonates i.e. pink above the ductus, blue below Pulse: absent/weak/delayed femorals, elevated BP in upper limbs; hyperdynamic neck pulsations Apex: thrusting Murmur: ejection systolic radiates through to the back
Pulmonary stenosis	Infancy: if severe, acute CCF, ± cyanosis due to right to left shunt via foramen ovale; otherwise asymptomatic in children Adult: CCF, arrhythmias	Jugular venous pulse: large 'a' wave; right ventricular heave Thrill: 2nd left interspace Heart sounds: soft 2nd Murmur: ejection click, then systolic ejection in 2nd interspace
Hypoplastic left heart	Few days old (2–6): CCF pale, severe acidosis like sepsis or an inborn error	Shock, low BP, death in days

Cyanotic congenital heart disease

	Age specific symptoms	Specific signs
Transposition of the great arteries	Cyanosis from birth or shortly after, proportional to shunt through foramen ovale, ductus arteriosus or a VSD. Breathless, CCF	Cyanosis, clubbing 100% oxygen: cyanosis not improved, may even worsen cyanosis by closing the ductus (= ductus dependent) Heart sounds: single Murmur: often absent *Chest X-ray: 'egg on side' heart shape
Fallot's tetralogy (pulmonary infundibular stenosis, VSD, right ventricle hypertrophies, aorta overrides	Infant: progressively deeper cyanosis, weeks or few months old. Cyanotic 'spells' from infundibular spasm Childhood: 'squatting' after exertion, SBE, cerebral abscesses, polycythaemia	Cyanosis, clubbing Right ventricular heave Heart sound: single 2nd Murmur: ejection systolic at 3rd left interspace *Chest X-ray: 'boot shaped' heart
Eisenmenger syndrome of irreversible pulmonary hypertension	Infant or child with VSD, transposition of the great arteries, PDA, or common atrioventricular canal in Down's syndrome. Torrential flow of blood through lungs causes the pulmonary vessels to thicken, irreversibly	Right parasternal (ventricular) heave and the pulmonary valve closing can be palpated Heart sound: loud pulmonary 2nd Murmur: ejection systolic ± early diastolic from pulmonary regurgitation

PDA = patent ductus arteriosus
* Classical finding present in only a half of cases

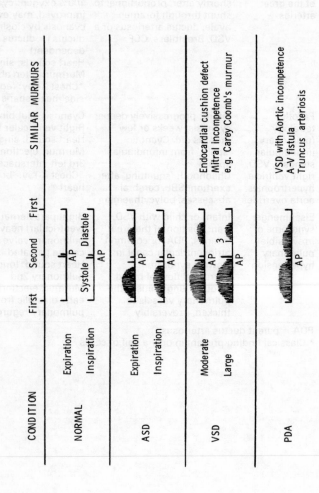

COMMONER AUSCULTATORY FINDINGS

(A = Aortic valve closure   P = pulmonary valve closure)

CONDITION		SIMILAR MURMURS
NORMAL	Expiration	
	Inspiration	
ASD	Expiration	
	Inspiration	
VSD	Moderate	Endocardial cushion defect Mitral incompetence e.g. Carey Coomb's murmur
	Large	
PDA		VSD with Aortic incompetence A-V fistula Truncus arteriosis

Fig. 17

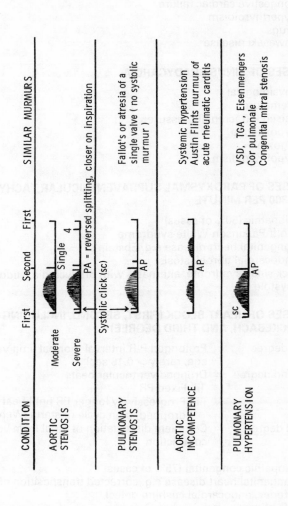

COMMONER AUSCULTATORY FINDINGS

(A = Aortic valve closure   P = Pulmonary valve closure)

CONDITION	First	Second	First	SIMILAR MURMURS
AORTIC STENOSIS	Moderate			
	Severe	Single 4		
		Systolic click (sc)	PA = reversed splitting, closer on inspiration	
PULMONARY STENOSIS		AP		Fallot's or atresia of a single valve (no systolic murmur)
AORTIC INCOMPETENCE		AP		Systemic hypertension Austin Flints murmur of acute rheumatic carditis
PULMONARY HYPERTENSION	sc	AP		VSD, TGA, Eisenmengers Cor pulmonale Congenital mitral stenosis

Fig. 18

CAUSES OF SINUS TACHYCARDIA

1. Fever
2. Anaemia
3. Hypovolaemia
4. Congestive cardiac failure
5. Hyperthyroidism
6. Drugs
7. Kawasaki disease

CAUSES OF SINUS BRADYCARDIA

1. Physiological
2. Premature
3. Raised intracranial pressure
4. Hypoxaemia
5. Digoxin
6. Hypothyroidism

CAUSES OF PAROXYSMAL SUPRAVENTRICULAR TACHYCARDIA, 200–300 PER MINUTE

1. Idiopathic (50% of cases)
2. Wolff-Parkinson-White syndrome
3. Congenital heart disease e.g. Ebstein's
4. Endocardial fibroelastosis
5. Sick sinus syndrome, alternates with bradycardia, sudden asystole

CAUSES OF HEART BLOCK (FIRST, SECOND, INCLUDING WENCKEBACH, AND THIRD DEGREE)

First degree   = Prolonged P-R interval (normal limit varies with age, rarely > 0.16 sec)

Second degree   = Dropped ventricular beats
  (i) Fixed PR
  (ii) Progressively longer PR until beat is dropped, then cycle re-starts (Wenckebach)

Third degree   = Complete dissociation of atrial from ventricular contraction

1. Idiopathic congenital (75% of cases)
2. Congenital heart disease e.g. corrected transposition of the great arteries, endocardial cushion defect
3. Infective
   (i) Bacterial e.g. diphtheria, coxsackie B
   (ii) Viral e.g. exanthema
4. Connective tissue
   (i) Acute rheumatic fever
   (ii) Maternal lupus (congenital heart block)

5. Endocardial fibroelastosis
6. Digoxin, hyperkalaemia
7. Intracardiac surgery
8. Familial

CAUSES OF VENTRICULAR PREMATURE BEATS

1. Physiological
2. Progression to ventricular tachycardia or fibrillation possible
   (i) Hypoxia, hyperkalaemia, hypercalcaemia
   (ii) Myocarditis
   (iii) Drugs: digoxin (bigeminy is characteristic), quinine, tricyclics (accidental ingestion)
   (iv) Jervell-Lange-Nielsen syndrome of familial congenital deafness and syncope, sudden death

CAUSES OF CARDIAC FAILURE

1. Stress: fever, hypoxia, infection, acidosis, hypoglycaemia
2. Anaemia, polycythaemia
3. Fluid overload
4. Thyrotoxicosis
5. Cardiac
   (i) Neonatal
      a. Volume overload: PDA, cardiac or cranial arterio-venous fistula
      b. Pressure overload: hypoplastic left heart, coarctation, total anomalous pulmonary venous drainage (TAPVD)
      c. Myocarditis: coxsackie B
      d. Arrhythmia: complete heart block
   (ii) Infancy
      a. Volume overload as pulmonary vascular resistance falls in the first weeks of life: VSD, single ventricle, TAPVD
      b. Pressure overload: pulmonary hypertension, pulmonary stenosis
      c. Myocarditis: endocardial fibroelastosis, infection e.g. mumps, Echo, Kawasaki disease
      d. Arrhythmia: paroxysmal supraventricular tachycardia
   (iii) Child: systemic hypertension, pulmonary hypertension (p. 97), bacterial endocarditis, myocarditis

CAUSES OF CYANOSIS

1. Depression of central nervous system: drugs, trauma, asphyxia
2. Seizures
3. Respiratory disease
4. Stress: septicaemia, hypoglycaemia, adrenal crisis
5. Polycythaemia in the newborn

6. Cardiac
   (i) Neonatal: transposition of the great arteries (TGA),
                      persistent fetal circulation, truncus arteriosus,
                      atresia or stenosis of pulmonary or tricuspid
                      valve, Ebstein's malformation of tricuspid
                      valve
   (ii) Infancy: Fallot's tetralogy, tricuspid atresia, Ebstein's,
                      TAPVD
   (iii) Child: Pulmonary hypertension (p. 97) —
                      Eisenmenger's syndrome
7. Methaemoglobinaemia

CAUSES OF RAISED BLOOD PRESSURE

Acute
1. Renal: acute glomerulonephritis, trauma
2. Burns
3. CNS: infection, space occupation
4. Haemolytic uraemic syndrome (p. 183)

Chronic
1. Renal: infected, scarred, obstructed and congenitally abnormal
   kidneys, tumours — Wilm's, neuroblastoma
2. Vascular: renal artery stenosis (neurofibromatosis), coarctation
   of the aorta
3. Endocrine: corticosteroids (including Cushing's syndrome), oral
   contraceptives, phaeochromocytoma, primary
   hyperaldosteronism (Conn's syndrome)
4. Miscellaneous: essential hypertension, obesity

CLINICAL CHARACTERISTICS OF SYSTEMIC JUVENILE CHRONIC ARTHRITIS (STILL'S DISEASE) RHEUMATIC FEVER AND HENOCH-SCHÖNLEIN (ANAPHYLACTOID) PURPURA

	Still's disease	Rheumatic fever	Henoch-Schönlein purpura
Cause	Autoimmune	BHS	BHS, viral, allergy
Age	1–5 years	4–7 years	>1 year, peak at 5 years.
Fever	Diurnal/any pattern	Sustained	Normal/raised
Rash	Maculopapular	E. marginatum	Urticarial/purpuric
Joints	Neck, knee, hip, foot, hand	Wrist, elbow knee, ankle	Wrist, ankle, knee
RES	Glands, hepatosplenomegaly	Liver++ if in heart failure	No enlargement
Heart	Pericarditis	Pericarditis and carditis	No involvement
Urine	Normal	Normal	Haematuria
Abdomen	Occasional pain	Normal	Acute pain common
Duration	Months	Days<weeks	Days>weeks

BHS = Beta Haemolytic streptococcus; RES = Reticulo-endothelial system

REVISED JONES CRITERIA FOR DIAGNOSIS OF RHEUMATIC PEVER

Major criteria
1. Arthritis
2. Carditis
3. Erythema marginatum
4. Subcutaneous nodules
5. Sydenham's chorea

Minor criteria
1. Previous history of rheumatic fever
2. Arthralgia
3. Elevated erythrocyte sedimentation rate (ESR)
4. Prolonged P-R interval on electrocardiogram
5. Fever

Evidence of streptococcal infection
1. Positive culture
2. Scarlet fever rash
3. Elevated antistreptolysin O antibodies (ASOT)

For diagnosis
Two major or 1 major + two Minor + evidence of preceding streptococcal infection

ELECTROCARDIOGRAPHY (ECG)

1. Normal change in vertical QRS axis with age (Fig. 19)
2. T-waves upright (positive) in V_4R, V_1 and V_2 up to 5 days old, or subsequently in left ventricular hypertrophy. Otherwise inverted (negative) until 6–12 years old
3. Changes in vertical QRS axis in some congenital malformations (Fig. 20)
4. Causes of selected ECG changes
     (i) Right ventricular hypertrophy in pulmonary stenosis, Fallot's tetralogy, pulmonary hypertension, transposition of the great arteries (TGA)
     (ii) Left ventricular hypertrophy in aortic stenosis and incompetence, VSD, PDA, coarctation, mitral regurgitation, cardiomyopathy, endocardial fibroelastosis
    (iii) Biventricular hypertrophy in large VSD
    (iv) Dextrocardia: inverted P-wave in I, aVR, upright in III. Normal looking chest leads in reverse order
     (v) ASD secundum: prolonged PR, RBBB pattern of rsR in V_1
    (vi) Endocardial cushion defect: negative QRS in I, aVF and RBBB
   (vii) Tricuspid atresia: negative QRS in I, aVF

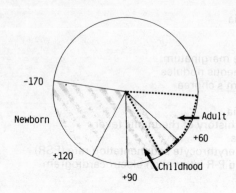

Fig. 19

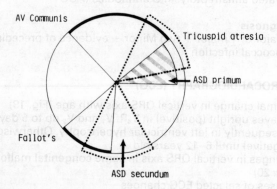

Fig. 20

(viii) Wolff Parkinson White syndrome: short PR, broad QRS with delta wave due to accessory aberrant conduction pathway

5. Selected ECG changes of ventricular hypertrophy
  (i) Biventricular hypertrophy = R + S in V_3 or V_4 > 70 mV
  (ii) Right ventricular hypertrophy
    a. less than 3 months old = R wave in V_4R > 15 mV
    b. more than 3 months old = R wave V_4R > 10 mV
  (iii) Left ventricular hypertrophy
    a. less than 3 months old = R wave in V_6 > 20 mV
    b. more than 3 months old = R wave in V_6 > 25 mV

6. Biochemical effects on the ECG
   (i) Hypokalaemia: arrhythmias, prolongs QT, depresses ST, prominent U-wave
   (ii) Hyperkalaemia: arrhythmias, elevates T wave, spreading of QRST
   (iii) Hypocalcaemia: prolongs QT
   (iv) Hypercalcaemia: shortens QT
7. Ischaemic changes in Kawasaki disease

RADIOLOGICAL FEATURES TO LOOK FOR

A. Normal
1. Cardiothoracic ratio (CTR) of 0.50 or less, except between 12 and 18 months, when the upper limit is 0.55
2. Thymus shadow may give impression of cardiomegaly, but sail shape or wave sign (p. 86) helps to discriminate. In cyanotic conditions the thymus rapidly involutes

B. Changes in pulmonary blood flow (PBF)
1. Cyanotic congenital heart disease

↓ PBF	↑ PBF
Fallot's tetralogy	Transposition of great arteries
Pulmonary atresia	Truncus arteriosus
Tricuspid atresia	Hypoplastic left heart
Ebstein's malformation	Single ventricle
	Total anomalous pulmonary venous drainage

2. Acyanotic congenital heart disease

Normal PBF	↑ PBF	↓ PBF
Coarctation	Atrial septal defect	Pulmonary stenosis
Aortic stenosis	Ventricular septal defect	Pulmonary hypertension (often 'pruned' look to bronchovascular markings)
	Patent ductus arteriosus	
	Arterio-venous fistula	

C. Cardiomegaly (CTR >0.5)
1. Congestive cardiac failure
2. Pericardial effusion
3. Myocarditis
4. Cardiomyopathy
5. Complete heart block
6. Ebstein's malformation

D. Absent pulmonary artery shadow
1. Severe pulmonary stenosis, atresia, in Fallot's tetralogy
2. Transposition of the great arteries, truncus arteriosus
3. Tricuspid atresia

E. Right-sided aortic arch
1. Normal
2. In 20% of children with Fallot's tetralogy
3. In transposition of the great arteries, truncus arteriosus, dextrocardia

F. Rib notching
Collateral circulation in coarctation of the aorta, rarely been before 5 years of age

RECOMMENDED READING

Shinebourne E A, Anderson R H 1980 Current paediatric cardiology. Oxford University Press, Oxford

Gastroenterology

EXAMINATION

1. Mouth: ask the child to show the teeth first, then to say 'ah' or 'eh'. Demonstration by a parent or attendant helps. Crying may reveal all! Alternatively, have the child held sat facing forward on parent's lap, one arm encircling the child's arms and upper trunk, the other hand restraining the forehead against the adult's chest. This hold also enables the ears to be inspected by rotating the head from side to side (p. 76).

   The buccal mucosa is inspected for Koplick's spots, thrush, torn frenulum from trauma, etc

2. Teeth: by the age of 2 years all 20 milk teeth should be present; eruption of the permanent teeth from 6 to 13 years, excluding third molars.

3. Gums: Asian and African children often have dark brown-blue pigmentation, with bluish pink interdental papillae, but the underside and edges of the tongue should be pink. At the gum margin a black line is seen in lead poisoning, but is also a normal finding in African children

4. Abdomen
   (i) Inspection. A thin abdominal wall with intestinal 'ladder' pattern is common in prematures and some term infants. The rectus muscles are often 1–2 cm apart (divarication of the recti) in infancy. Umbilical hernias reduce easily, rarely obstruct and generally resolve by 2 years, or 5 years in Africans who also tend to have a pot-bellied appearance owing to a physiological lumbar lordosis
   (ii) Palpation
   The liver (hatched area) is a large abdominal organ crossing the midline. Place the right hand gently on the abdomen from the child's right side, and using the radial side of the index finger to feel for the liver edge, advance from the groin, hand parallel to the right costal margin. Percuss along the same line of advance to confirm size. Normal values are 3 cm below the costal margin in the nipple line in infancy, 2 cm at 1 year and 1 cm at 5 years.

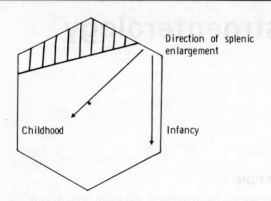

Fig. 21

The spleen is palpable in normal infants though seldom more than 1 cm, and occasionally in health after 1 year old, although it frequently enlarges during infections (p. 120). It is smooth in outline at first, becoming notched in later childhood.

The kidneys are lower in infants than children and easily palpated, and fetal lobulation may be felt. In the neonate, flex the thighs with one hand, and with the other palpate the kidneys with the thumb in a gentle pincer action against the fingers of that hand, which slip under the back to support it. The right kidney is lower than the left, and both move headwards on expiration.

The bladder is often palpable in early childhood as it is an intra-abdominal organ. Ensure it disappears on voiding, especially in boys, to help exclude outlet obstruction

CAUSES OF COMMONER SWELLINGS IN THE NECK (Fig. 22)

Midline
1. Submandibular lymph gland
2. Dermoid cyst, attached to the skin, not deeper structures like '3'
3. Thyroglossal cyst, moves upwards on protrusion of tongue
4. Thyroid gland, moves upwards on swallowing

Lateral
A. Cystic hygroma, usually in the posterior triangle of the neck from birth
B. Sternomastoid tumour, causing torticollis, from 2 weeks old
C. Parotid gland
D. Jugulo-digastric lymph gland. Position of the swelling above (C) or below (D), the angle of the jaw differentiates C and D

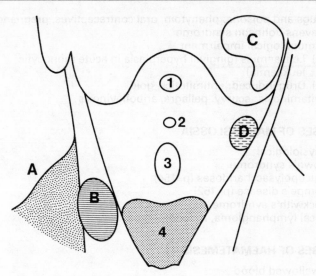

Fig. 22

CAUSES OF UMBILICAL HERNIA

1. Physiological, especially African
2. Prematures
3. Down's syndrome
4. Hypothyroidism
5. Mucopolysaccharidoses

CAUSES OF INGUINAL SWELLINGS

1. Enlarged lymph glands
2. Inguinal hernia
3. Hydrocoele (causes confusion, and inguinal hernia may be associated with it)
4. Undescended testis

CAUSES OF GINGIVOSTOMATITIS

1. Infection:
   (i) Viruses: measles, primary herpes simplex, Coxsackie A (herpangina, hand, foot and mouth disease)
   (ii) Bacteria: streptococcus, diphtheria, Vincent's angina, noma
   (iii) Fungal: monilia
2. Aphthous ulcers: alone, with coeliac disease
3. Local reaction: mouth washes, cheek biting, aspirin

4. Drugs and poisons: phenytoin, oral contraceptives, pregnancy
5. Stevens-Johnson syndrome
6. Immunological impairment
   (i) Leukaemias (gingival hyperplasia in acute monocytic leukaemia)
   (ii) Drug induced: antimitotics, gold
7. Avitaminosis: scurvy, pellagra, ariboflavinosis

CAUSES OF MACROGLOSSIA

1. Physiological
2. Down's syndrome
3. Mucopolysaccharidoses (p. 154)
4. Pompe's disease (p. 152)
5. Beckwith's syndrome
6. Local lymphangioma, rhabdomyoma

CAUSES OF HAEMATEMESIS

1. Swallowed blood
   (i) Neonate: maternal, at birth or cracked nipple
   (ii) Epistaxis
2. Vomiting repeatedly, acute gastritis
3. Ulceration
   (i) Hiatus hernia
   (ii) Drugs: aspirin, iron poisoning
   (iii) Peptic ulcer
   (iv) Foreign body
4. Munchausen by proxy (factitious bleeding)
5. Rare but important: oesophageal varices, bleeding disorders (p. 129), vascular malformations e.g. haemangioma, telangiectasia, arterio-venous malformations
N.B. Exclude colourings as a cause first

CAUSES OF PROJECTILE VOMITING

1. Urinary tract infection
2. Pyloric stenosis
3. Duodenal stenosis or atresia, duodenal ulcer
4. Malrotation of the bowel
5. Raised intracranial pressure
6. Cow's milk protein intolerance
7. Adrenal insufficiency

CLINICAL FEATURES OF HIATUS HERNIA VERSUS PYLORIC STENOSIS

	Hiatus hernia	Pyloric stenosis
Age at onset	First week	2–6 weeks
Sex	Males = Females	Firstborn males (M:F = 5:1)
Family history	—	In 20%
Vomiting	Continuous, wells up, fresh/altered blood if ulceration present; no bile	Forceful, soon after feeds; altered blood occasionally; no bile
Nutrition	Slowly progressive failure to thrive; repeated aspiration and pneumonia occur	Acute weight loss, dehydration, metabolic acidosis
Stools	Occasionally constipated, altered blood	Starvation stools

N.B. Feeding mismanagement and urinary infections share many of these symptoms and signs

ABDOMINAL EXAMINATION IN PYLORIC STENOSIS

Inspection: visible peristalsis, moving transversely from the left upper quadrant downwards towards the midline above the umbilicus
Palpation: from the baby's left hand side place the palm of your left hand on the abdomen with fingers curling round the lateral edge of the right rectus muscle midway between the lower edge of the rib cage and the level of the umbilicus. The pylorus muscle is towards the back, contracts into a rubbery pea shape then relaxes ('have I lost it?'), only to harden up again, every few minutes

CAUSES OF VOMITING

1. Non-organic
   (i) Infants: overfeeding, posseting, rumination
   (ii) Children: self-induced, overeating
   (iii) Adolescents: anorexia/bulimia nervosa
2. Infection: gastroenteritis or as parenteral response to urine infection, otitis media etc
3. Gastrointestinal disorders
   (i) Medical: hiatus hernia, food allergies (cow's milk protein intolerance), coeliac disease
   (ii) Surgical: pyloric stenosis, acute obstruction, appendicitis; repeated episodes may occur in malrotation

4. Cough: pertussis, asthma
5. Migraine, cyclical vomiting
6. Medication: emetics, valproate, flucloxacillin
7. Uncommon but important
   (i) Metabolic: diabetes mellitus, uraemia, congenital adrenal hyperplasia
   (ii) Raised intracranial pressure

CAUSES OF PALPABLE ABDOMINAL MASSES

Neonatal (see p. 25)

Infancy and childhood

1. Renal: hydronephrosis, Wilms' tumour, multicystic and polycystic disease
2. GIT
   (i) Duplications
   (ii) Pyloric stenosis
   (iii) Intussusception under right lobe of liver
   (iv) Right iliac fossa: appendicitis abscess, intussusception, tuberculosis Crohn's, amoebiasis, leukaemia, ovarian tumour, ectopic kidney
3. Hepatosplenomegaly (p. 120)
   (i) Infective
   (ii) Haematological
   (iii) Malignancy
   (iv) Congestive cardiac failure
   (v) Cirrhosis
   (vi) Storage diseases
4. Malignancy: leukaemia, neuroblastoma, lymphoma, teratoma, sarcoma
5. Miscellaneous: choledochal cyst, Fallopian tube and ovarian torsion

CAUSES OF ABDOMINAL DISTENSION

Neonatal (see p. 24)

Infancy and childhood

1. Air swallowing: feeding, habit, tracheo-oesophageal fistula
2. Intestinal
   (i) Peritonitis, paralytic ileus, acute obstruction
   (ii) Dysentery
   (iii) Coeliac disease
   (iv) Meconium ileus equivalent in cystic fibrosis
   (v) Hirschsprung's disease
   (vi) Faecal Impaction, inspirated curds
   (vii) Crohn's, ulcerative colitis
   (viii) Hypokalaemia

3. Ascites
   (i) Congestive cardiac failure
   (ii) Nephrotic syndrome
   (iii) Acute glomerulonephritis
   (iv) Malnutrition
   (v) Malignancy
   (vi) Cirrhosis
   (vii) Protein losing enteropathy
4. Abdominal masses: renal, GIT, hepatosplenomegaly, malignancies

COMMON CAUSES OF ACUTE ABDOMINAL PAIN

Medical (exclude coughing)
1. Infection: gastroenteritis, 'mesenteric adenitis', lower lobe pneumonia, urinary tract infection, acute hepatitis
2. Constipation
3. Henoch-Schonlein (Anaphylactoid) purpura
4. Acute nephritis
5. Rare but important e.g. diabetes mellitus, sickle cell crisis, Kawasaki disease, lead poisoning

Surgical
1. Acute appendicitis
2. Obstruction: intussusception, strangulated inguinal hernia, volvulus
3. Renal: hydronephrosis, colic
4. Torsion of testis or ovary

COMMON CAUSES OF ACUTE ABDOMINAL PAIN BY AGE

At all ages
Acute gastroenteritis: viral, bacterial, parasitic (p. 116)

Infancy
1. Surgical
   (i) Strangulated hernia
   (ii) Intussusception
   (iii) Volvulus/obstruction of the bowel
   (iv) Appendicitis
   (v) Hirschsprung's disease
   (vi) Testicular torsion
   (vii) Meckel's diverticulitis
2. Medical
   (i) Urinary tract infection
   (ii) Pneumonia
   (iii) Trauma, non-accidental
   (iv) Cow's milk protein and lactose intolerance
   (v) Rare: lead poisoning, porphyria

Childhood
1. Psychological/migraine (p. 75)
2. Infective
   (i) Mesenteric adenitis
   (ii) Acute hepatitis, infectious mononucleosis
   (iii) Urinary tract infection
   (iv) Pneumonia
   (v) Rare: pancreatitis
3. Surgical
   (i) Appendicitis
   (ii) Trauma to bowel, spleen etc
   (iii) Rare: Meckel's diverticulitis, testicular torsion
4. Miscellaneous
   (i) Constipation
   (ii) Food allergy, lactose intolerance
   (iii) Henoch-Schönlein anaphylactoid purpura
   (iv) Peptic ulcer
   (v) Sickle cell viruses
   (vi) Ulcerative colitis
   (vii) Diabetes mellitus, hypoglycaemia
5. Gynaecological (adolescent)
   (i) Menstruation
   (ii) Pelvic inflamatory disease
   (iii) Ovarian cyst
   (iv) Ectopic pregnancy
   (v) Haematocolpos

RECURRENT ABDOMINAL PAIN

Three discrete episodes of abdominal pain in a 3 month period, interfering with regular activities and school attendance; it affects 10% of school children

CLINICAL FEATURES OF APPENDICITIS VERSUS MESENTERIC ADENITIS

	Appendicitis	Mesenteric adenitis
Recurrent	—	Previous episodes common
Upper respiratory tract infection	Maybe	Within 24 hours, cervical glands +
Temperature and appearance	Usually 38°C, in pre-school up to 40°C, ill, becomes toxic	39–40°C common, flushed
Vomiting	Frequent	Unusual
Abdominal tenderness, guarding	Marked, usually very distressed, localised to right side, young child pushes hand away + +	Vague generalised, periumbilical, often comes and goes
Rectal examination	Localised tenderness on right	No localised tenderness

CAUSES OF RECURRENT ABDOMINAL PAIN

1. Migrainous or psychological stress in 95%
2. Mesenteric adenitis
3. Constipation
4. Food allergy, lactose intolerance
5. GIT.: peptic ulcer, constipation, worms, Crohn's disease, ulcerative colitis
6. Renal: hydronephrosis, recurrent pyelonephritis, calculi
7. Metabolic: ketotic diabetes mellitus, hypoglycaemia, lead, hypercholesterolaemia, porphyria
8. Pancreatitis
9. Epilepsy
10. Referred pain from spine, chest, etc

CAUSES OF CARBOHYDRATE MALABSORPTION

Confirmation
Solid stool is not suitable so that collection is made by placing the baby on plastic and the stool-water: water mix of 1:2 is tested using Clinitest. More than 0.5 per cent sugar is a positive result
1. Secondary disccharidase deficiency, usually lactase
    (i) Infective gastroenteritis, giardiasis
    (ii) Coeliac disease
    (iii) Prematurity
    (iv) Protein energy malnutrition (PEM)
    (v) Cow's milk protein intolerance

   (vi) Immune deficiency
  (vii) Drugs: Neomycin, Kanamycin
 (viii) Massive intestinal resection
2. Primary disaccharidase deficiency
    (i) Congenital alactasia, sucrase-isomaltase
   (ii) Progressive deficiency mainly in non-Caucasian adults,
        especially of African origin
3. Monosaccharide deficiency
    (i) Secondary to PEM, gastroenteritis, neonatal bowel
        surgery, hypogammaglobulinaemia
   (ii) Primary congenital glucose — galactose malabsorption
        (rare)

CAUSES OF ACUTE DIARRHOEA

1. Starvation stools (mucousy, watery and green)
2. Infection: rota and enterovirus, *Escherichia coli*, shigella,
   salmonella, campylobacter, giardia, amoeba, yersinia
3. Food poisoning toxins: staphylococcal
4. Parenteral response to infection e.g. pneumonia, otitis media etc
5. Surgical: pelvic appendicitis, intussusception, Hirschsprung's
   disease
6. Drugs: laxatives, directly or via breast milk, antibiotics
7. Prodrome to haemolytic uraemia syndrome, haemorrhagic
   shock encephalopathy syndrome, Kawasaki disease, toxic shock
   syndrome

CAUSES OF CHRONIC DIARRHOEA

1. Failure to gain weight, or actual weight loss, and persistent
   loose watery stools for more than 2 weeks
    (i) Enteric infections: see above; note that immuno-deficiency
        may be present
   (ii) Post-enteric infection: lactose and cow's milk protein
        intolerance, transient gluten enteropathy
  (iii) Inflammatory bowel disease: food allergies, ulcerative
        colitis, Crohn's disease
   (iv) Malabsorption: coeliac disease, cystic fibrosis
2. Normal growth, loose or semiformed stools
    (i) Chronic non-specific toddler's diarrhoea
   (ii) Constipation with overflow
  (iii) Laxative abuse, a form of Munchausen by proxy or
        bulimia nervosa in older child

Rare causes of diarrhoea in infancy and childhood
1. Immuno-deficiency
   (i) IgA deficiency, transient hypo γ globulinaemia
   (ii) Severe combined immuno-deficiency (SCID)
   (iii) Opsonisation defect
   (iv) Di George's syndrome
   (v) Wiskott-Aldrich syndrome
   (vi) Pancreatic insufficiency with cyclic neutropenia
2. Tumour: neuroblastoma, ganglioneuroma, Zollinger-Ellison syndrome
3. Malabsorption: abetalipoproteinaemia, Wolman's disease, intestinal lymphangiectasia
4. Acrodermatitis enteropathica
5. Congenital: chloridorrhoea, enterokinase deficiency, bile salt deficiency

CAUSES OF A FLAT SMALL INTESTINAL MUCOSA

1. Coeliac disease
2. Gastroenteritis
3. Giardiasis
4. Intolerance of cow's milk, soy protein
5. Protein energy malnutrition
6. Hypo γ globulinaemia

CAUSES OF A SWEAT SODIUM OF 70 mmol/l OR MORE

1. Cystic fibrosis
2. Technical errors: insufficient weight of sweat, salt from fingers or environment contaminating filter paper or equipment
3. Metabolic: glucose-6-phosphatase deficiency, adrenal insufficiency, nephrogenic diabetes insipidus, mucopolysaccharidoses
4. Insufficient sweat: hypothyroidism, ectodermal dysplasia, Riley-Day syndrome
5. Malnutrition

CHARACTERISTICS OF CYSTIC FIBROSIS AND COELIAC DISEASE

	Cystic fibrosis	Coeliac (untreated)
Newborn	Meconium ileus	—
Infant	Failure to thrive from birth; recurrent pneumonia	Failure to thrive from introduction of gluten, usually at 3–4 months old
1. Stools	Often abnormal from birth, diarrhoeal, very smelly, oily like melted butter	Normal until gluten introduced; become pale and bulky; not oily
2. Appetite	Voracious	Poor
3. Chest	'Bronchitis' frequent, i.e. recurrent bronchopneumonia	Normal
4. Social	Lively	Withdrawn, 'difficult'
5. Others	Rectal prolapse, salty taste to skin, heat exhaustion	Anaemia, rickets, long eyelashes
Child		
As above plus:		
1. Height	Relatively preserved	Short
2. Puberty	Delayed, males sterile	Delayed, amenorrhoea common in girls
3. Abdomen	Meconium ileus equivalent; biliary cirrhosis and portal hypertension cause enlarged spleen and oesophageal varices	Distended, liver edge not palpable, wasted buttocks
4. Others	Cor pulmonale; nasal polyps; diabetes mellitus	School failure from lethargy
Screening	Neonatal blood trypsin level elevated (Guthrie card may be used)	One hour after oral D-xylose, blood level <20 mg/100 ml (not 100% reliable)
Diagnosis	Sweat sodium 70 mmol/l or more on at least 100 mg of sweat	Villous atrophy, heals on diet, relapses on gluten i.e. 3 jejunal biopsies

CAUSES OF CONSTIPATION

1. Starvation, dehydration
2. Obstruction, paralytic ileus
3. Voluntary: encopresis, anal fissure
4. Neurological: hypotonia, cerebral palsy, mental retardation, spina bifida
5. Metabolic: rickets, hypothyroidism, hypercalcaemia, lead poisoning

CAUSES OF ENCOPRESIS

1. Untrained
2. Confused training
3. Potty battle
4. Neurotic retention
5. Antisocial soiling
6. Sexual abuse
7. Psychotic

CAUSES OF COLORECTAL BLEEDING (exclude coloured drinks, dyes, beetroot)

1. Constipation, anal fissure
2. Swallowed blood
3. Dysentery and salmonellosis
4. Ulceration: hiatus hernia, peptic ulcer, Meckel's diverticulum, intestinal duplication, aspirin
5. Cow's milk protein intolerance
6. Intussusception
7. Henoch-Schönlein anaphylactoid purpura
8. Ulcerative colitis, Crohn's disease
9. Bleeding diathesis: haematological, uraemic, haemolytic–uraemic syndrome (p. 183)
10. Rare: polyps, portal hypertension, malignancy, Zollinger–Ellison syndrome
11. Münchhausen by proxy (p. 170)

CAUSES OF HEPATOMEGALY BY AGE OF ONSET

Neonatal
1. Infection: congenital, intrapartum, septicaemia, abscess
2. Haematological: haemolytic disease of the newborn
3. Congestive cardiac failure
4. Traumatic subcapsular haematoma
5. Biliary atresia
6. Neonatal hepatitis

Infancy and early childhood
1. Infection
   (i) Bacterial: septicaemia, brucellosis, tuberculosis, leptospirosis, syphilis
   (ii) Viral: infective hepatitis, infectious mononucleosis, cytomegalovirus
   (iii) Protozoal: malaria, toxoplasmosis, amoeba
   (iv) Parasites: hydatid, ascariasis
   (v) Fungal: histoplasmosis
2. Haematological: sickle cell, thalassaemia
3. Congestive cardiac failure

4. Cystic fibrosis
5. Malignancy
    (i) Leukaemia, Letterer-Siwe disease
    (ii) Metastatic: neuroblastoma, Wilms', ganodal
    (iii) Primary, e.g. hepatoma
6. Metabolic
    (i) Reye's syndrome
    (ii) Storage diseases e.g. glycogenoses (p. 152), mucopolysaccharidoses (p. 154), neurolipidoses (p. 153) Wolman's disease
    (iii) Galactosaemia, alpha-1-antitrypsin deficiency
7. Poisons and drugs
8. Portal hypertension

Older children and adolescents
1. Infection: as above
2. Chronic active hepatitis
3. Chronic inflammatory disease: Still's, ulcerative colitis, Crohn's
4. Lymphoma
5. Metabolic: Wilson's disease, alpha-1-antitrypsin deficiency, hepatic porphyria
6. Congenital hepatic fibrosis, polycystic liver disease
7. Amyloidosis

CAUSES OF SPLENOMEGALY

1. Infection
    (i) See hepatomegaly
    (ii) Bacterial endocarditis
    (iii) Kala-azar, schistosomiasis
2. Haematological
    (i) Haemolytic anaemias: sickle cell, HbC, thalassaemia, spherocytosis
    (ii) Severe iron deficiency anaemia
    (iii) Thrombocytopenia
3. Malignancy: lymphomas, lymphosarcoma, leukaemia, Letterer-Siwe disease
4. Portal hypertension
5. Miscellaneous: storage diseases, Still's disease, amyloidosis, Banti's syndrome

CAUSES OF HEPATOSPLENOMEGALY

1. Infection: hepatitis A and B, infectious mononucleosis, malaria, septicaemia
2. Haematological: mainly spleen in spherocytosis, sickle cell, severe iron deficiency anaemia, thrombocytopenia
3. Congestive cardiac failure, mainly liver

4. Malignancy: leukaemia, lymphoma, secondary deposits in the liver e.g. neuroblastoma
5. Rare: portal hypertension, storage disorders, polycystic liver disease

Causes of portal hypertension in childhood
1. Pre-sinusoidal
   (i) Extrahepatic: portal vein thrombosis, e.g. umbilical vein sepsis, exchange tranfusions, polycythaemia
   (ii) Intrahepatic: congenital hepatic fibrosis, infiltrations, schistosomiasis
2. Post-sinusoidal
   (i) Extrahepatic: hepatic vein thrombosis (Budd-Chiari), congestive cardiac failure, constrictive cardiac failure
   (ii) Intrahepatic: cirrhosis, veno-occlusive disease (bush teas)

CAUSES OF JAUNDICE IN INFANTS AND CHILDREN

Neonatal (see p. 21)

Unconjugated
1. Haemolytic: spherocytosis, thalassaemia, sickle cell disease glucose-6-phosphatase deficiency
2. Metabolic: Gilbert's, Crigler-Najjar, erythropoietic porphyria

Conjugated > 25 μmol/l (1.5 mg/100 ml)
1. Infection
   (i) Viruses e.g. hepatitis A and B, infectious mononucleosis, cytomegalovirus
   (ii) Bacteria e.g. septicaemia, urinary tract infection, leptospirosis
   (iii) Protozoa e.g. malaria, toxoplasmosis
   (iv) Miscellaneous e.g. toxocara, trichinella, ascaris
2. Drugs
   (i) Cholestatic e.g. phenothiazines, anabolic steroids, erythromycin estolate
   (ii) Hepatocellular, e.g. poisoning by paracetamol, iron, CCl_4, antithyroid drugs, halothane, isoniazid, rifampicin
3. Metabolic
   (i) Wilson's disease, galactosaemia, fructosaemia, tryosinosis
   (ii) Cystic fibrosis, alpha-1-antitrypsin deficiency
   (iii) Storage diseases e.g. glycogenesis type, IV, Niemann-Pick
   (iv) Dubin-Johnson, Rotor syndrome
4. Chronic inflammatory: chronic active hepatitis, Crohn's, ulcerative colitis
5. Biliary obstruction: extrahepatic, intrahepatic biliary atresia, choledochal cyst, gallstones

CAUSES OF RADIO-OPACITIES ON ABDOMINAL X-RAY

1. Bowel
   - (i) Foreign body, iron tablets, faecoliths
   - (ii) Meconium peritonitis, tuberculous peritonitis or lymph glands
2. Renal: calculi, tubular necrosis, medullary cystic disease
3. Adrenal: calcification after neonatal shock, Addison's disease, Wolman's disease
4. Liver
   - (i) Amoebic or hydatid cyst, tuberculosis, haemangioma, hepatoma
   - (ii) Intrahepatic biliary calculi, gallbladder calculi
5. Bladder: calculi, foreign body, schistosomiasis
6. Muscle
   - (i) Abdominal wall: myositis ossificans, cysterci
   - (ii) Psoas: cysterci
7. Tumour: neuroblastoma, nephroblastoma, dermoid, teratoma

WHEN PRESENTED WITH A NEONATAL X-RAY CONSIDER THE FOLLOWING

1. Situs inversus
2. Double bubble of duodenal atresia. Also seen with annular pancreas, malrotation of mid-gut with volvulus, Ladd's bands
3. Fluid levels: ileal atresia, meconium ileus, meconium plug syndrome, atresia of colon, small left colon syndrome, Hirschsprung's disease
4. Intraluminal gas (double wall to bowel): necrotising enterocolitis
5. Fluid levels and 'bubbles' in the bowel: meconium ileus
6. Calcification flecks: meconium peritonitis
7. Inverted lateral of abdomen and hips, with radio-opaque anal marker; consider ano-rectal atresia
8. Spinal anomalies: gross spina bifida, sacral agenesis, remembering that the spinous processes of the affected vertebral bodies are usually *not* seen
9. Congenital dislocation of hip(s)

FURTHER READING

O'Donnell B 1985 Abdominal pain in children. Blackwell Oxford
Tripp J H, Candy D C A 1985 Manual of paediatric gastroenterology. Churchill Livingstone, Edinburgh
Walker-Smith J A, Hamilton J R, Walker W A 1983 Practical paediatric gastroenterology. Butterworths, London

Haematology

NORMAL CHANGES IN HAEMATOLOGY

	Haemoglobin Hb g/dl	Packed cell volume (PCV)	Mean corpuscular volume (MCV)
Birth	19	60	120
6–10 weeks	11	35	100
1–10 years	12	40	80
Adolescence	14	40	90

Iron stores: At birth mainly in circulating haemoglobin
Haemoglobin: At birth, HbF = 50–80%, Adult HbA = 15–40%
HbA$_2$ and methaemoglobin each < 1% of total.
HbF 5% at six months, < 2% by 3 years

LEUCOCYTES

1. At birth 9 to 30 × 10^9/1, 6–8 × 10^9/1 to one year, 5–15 × 10^9/1 thereafter
2. Lymphocyte preponderance from 3 weeks to 9 years
3. Neutropenia $\Big\}$ = < 1.5 × 10^9/1 at any age
4. Lymphopenia

CAUSES OF A LOW MCV

Microcytic anaemia due to
1. Iron deficiency $\Big\}$ reduced RBC count
2. Lead poisoning
3. Thalassaemia minor: normal RBC count
4. Protein energy malnutrition
5. Chronic inflammation, e.g. Still's disease
6. Rare: sideroblastic anaemia, copper deficiency

CAUSES OF NORMOCYTIC ANAEMIA

1. Decreased production (see normochromic anaemia, p. 126)
2. Haemolytic anaemias (p. 127)
3. Acute blood loss (p. 127)

CAUSES OF MACROCYTOSIS (HIGH MCV)

1. Normal: newborn
2. Reticulocytes (are macrocytes): haemolysis, haemorrhage
3. Metabolic: protein energy malnutrition, hypothyroidism, cirrhosis
4. Vitamin: folate deficiency, B12 deficiency, scurvy
5. Miscellaneous: Down's syndrome, leukaemia, congenital RBC aplasia, hereditary orotic aciduria (very rare)

CAUSES OF A HIGH MEAN CORPUSCULAR HAEMOGLOBIN CONCENTRATION (MCHC)

Spherocytosis
1. Hereditary spherocytosis
2. ABO incompatibility
3. Auto-immune haemolytic anaemia
4. Haemolytic uraemic syndrome

CAUSES OF HYPOCHROMIC ANAEMIA

Condition		Serum concentration	
	Iron	Ferritin	Total iron binding capacity
Iron deficiency	↓	↓	↑
Chronic infection or inflammation	↓	↑	N
Thalassaemia	↑	↑ ↑	N

Rare: sideroblastic anaemia, pulmonary haemosiderosis, congenital transferase deficiency, copper deficiency

CAUSES OF TARGET CELLS

1. Thalassaemia
2. Haemoglobinopathy: sickle cell disease, HbC, HbSC etc
3. Iron deficiency anaemia
4. Lead poisoning
5. Liver disease, jaundice
6. Splenectomy

CAUSES OF RED CELL INCLUSION BODIES

1. Heinz body anaemia: denatured haemoglobin particles in reticulocytes
   (i) Prematurity, related to high HbF content
   (ii) Glucose-6-phosphate dehydrogenase deficiency
   (iii) Haemolytic anaemia due to drugs (p. 128)
   (iv) Unstable haemoglobins e.g. HbH
2. Howell-Jolly bodies: nuclear remnants in red cells
   (i) Thalassaemia major
   (ii) Post splenectomy
3. Punctate basophilia
   (i) Lead poisoning

CAUSES OF NEUTROPENIA

1. Decreased production
   (i) Infection: viruses, typhoid, brucella
   (ii) Irradiation, drugs e.g. chloramphenicol, antithyroid, anticonvulsant drugs
   (iii) Infiltration: leukaemia, tumour
   (iv) Rare:
      a. Nutritional: folate and B_{12} deficiency
      b. Severe combined immuno-deficiency
      d. Chronic neutropenia
      e. Shwachman's syndrome
2. Increased destruction
   (i) Drug induced immune neutropenia: any, but especially penicillins, sulphonamides
   (ii) Hypersplenism
   (iii) Auto-immune: juvenile rheumatoid arthritis, connective tissue disease
   (iv) Iso-immune
      a. Neonatal from mother
      b. Idiopathic

CAUSES OF LEUCOCYTOSIS

1. Physiological (p. 123)
2. Infection
3. Trauma, bleeding, burns
4. Acute hypoxia, especially in newborn, asthma
5. Metabolic: diabetes mellitus, renal failure
6. Malignancy, leukaemia

CAUSES OF LYMPHOCYTOSIS

1. Physiological
2. Infection
    (i) Atypical lymphocytes: infectious mononucleosis, cytomegalovirus
    (ii) Acute infectious lymphocytosis, influenza, exanthemata, infective hepatitis
    (iii) Bacterial infections in children, particularly pertussis, typhoid, brucellosis, rarely tuberculosis
3. Leukaemia
4. Still's disease

CAUSES OF ANAEMIA: DECREASED PRODUCTION, HAEMOLYSIS, BLOOD LOSS

A. Decreased production
1. Early dilutional anaemia of prematurity at 6–8 weeks
2. Hypochromic
    (i) Iron deficiency: dietary lack (p. 129), infection, blood loss, chronic inflammation
    (ii) Copper or pyridoxine deficiency
3. Normochromic
    (i) Chronic infection or inflammation
    (ii) Nutritional: protein energy malnutrition, scurvy
    (iii) Infiltration e.g. leukaemia, malignancy, tuberculosis
    (iv) Metabolic: cirrhosis, uraemia
    (v) Endocrine: hypothyroidism, hypopituitarism, hypoadrenal
4. Megaloblastic
    (i) Folic acid e.g. infection, coeliac, anticonvulsants, haemolysis
    (ii) B_{12} deficiency: coeliac, intestinal resections, Crohn's disease, juvenile PA
5. Hypoplastic (p. 129) e.g. crises, drugs, infiltration, congenital, etc

B. Haemolytic (see p. 127 for cause by age)
1. Membrane defects: spherocytosis, elliptocytosis, stomatocytosis, erythropoietic porphyria, a-betalipoproteinaemia
2. Haemoglobinopathies: haemoglobin S, thalassaemia major, etc
3. Enzyme deficiencies
    (i) Drug induced and spontaneous in glucose-6-phosphate dehydrogenase deficiency (p. 128)
    (ii) Glutathione synthesis, pyruvate kinase deficiency
4. Immune
    (i) Rhesus, ABO, blood transfusion
    (ii) Autoimmune e.g. reticuloses, methyl dopa, penicillin, mycoplasma, SLE

5. Non-immune: drugs, infection, splenomegaly, burns, haemolytic uraemic syndrome, DIC, vitamin E deficiency, porphyria, venoms

C. Blood loss
1. Perinatal
   (i) Placental and cord accidents
   (ii) Feto-maternal, feto-fetal transfusion
   (iii) Birth injury e.g. cephalhaematoma, bruising
   (iv) Haemorrhagic disease of the newborn
2. Epistaxis
3. Trauma: accidental, non-accidental
4. Alimentary tract: haematemesis (p. 110), rectal bleeding (p. 119)
5. Haematuria (p. 144)
6. Blood disorders e.g. haemophilia, thrombocytopenia, anaphylactoid purpura etc

CAUSES OF HAEMOLYTIC ANAEMIA, BY AGE AT PRESENTATION
1. Neonatal
   (i) Acquired
      a. Immune: rhesus, ABO
      b. Infection, congenital (TORCH p. 21), and acquired
   (ii) Genetic
      a. Enzyme deficiency e.g. glucose-6-phosphate dehydrogenase deficiency (G-6-PD) — sex-linked, Mediterranean, Asian and Black populations mainly affected. Haemolysis is spontaneous in newborn; later episodes precipitated by drugs, fava beans and sepsis
      b. Spherocytosis — autosomal dominant, large spleen, jaundice and anaemia, gall stones in adults
2. Infancy
   (i) Infection, acute e.g. septicaemia, malaria. Meningococcaemia may cause disseminated intravascular coagulation
   (ii) Genetic: sickle cell disease and thalassaemia both become manifest from 6 months as HbF production falls
   (iii) Haemolytic uraemic syndrome (p. 183)
3. Childhood
   (i) Acquired
      a. Infection, acute: see 2 (i) above
      b. Autoimmune Coomb's positive anaemia after infections e.g. mycoplasma, viral; also idiopathic, or may be drug induced
      c. Drugs e.g. penicillin, sulpha, nitrofurantoin
   (ii) Genetic
      Sickle cell disease, thalassaemia, spherocytosis, G-6-PD

CAUSES OF HAEMOLYTIC ANAEMIA DUE TO CHEMICALS, DRUGS, PLANTS AND VENOMS

1. Drugs
     (i) Hereditary enzyme deficiency
         a. Glucose-6-phosphate dehydrogenase
             Fava bean
             Antimalarials
             Sulphonamides
             Nitrofurans
             Antipyretics, but not aspirin
             Analgesics
             Vitamin K (water soluble analogue)
             (NB also infections and diabetic ketoacidosis)
         b. Reduced glutathione (GSH)
             GSH reductase, GSH synthetase, GSH peroxidase
             Antimalarials, etc
     (ii) Immunological: methyl dopa, phenacetin, quinidine, PAS, penicillin, sulphonamides
2. Inorganic chemicals: lead chlorates, arsenic
3. Venoms: snake, spider, bee
4. Plants: male fern, mushroom

CAUSES OF 'DEFICIENCY' ANAEMIAS

Up to 6 months old
1. Iron deficiency
     (i) Nutritional: premature infants, multiple births, delayed weaning (at least 4 months old)
     (ii) Infection
     (iii) Blood loss: perinatal — feto-maternal, feto-fetal transfusion, placental abruption, placenta praevia, iatrogenic after exchange transfusion (low PCV of donor blood)
     (iv) Maternal iron deficiency
2. Folic acid: prematures at 6–18 weeks
3. Thyroxine
4. Vitamin C: scurvy in prematures
5. Vitamin E: prematures, very low birth weight, at 6 to 12 weeks
6. Rare
     (i) Pyridoxine: familial and sporadic
     (ii) Copper: premature infants and prolonged intravenous alimentation.

Over 6 months old
1. Iron deficiency
     (i) Nutritional
     (ii) Malabsorption: coeliac, cow's milk protein intolerance

(iii) Blood loss: haematemesis (p. 110), rectal bleeding (p. 119), haematuria (p. 144), epistaxis, menses
(iv) Adolescent growth spurt
2. Folic acid
  (i) Malabsorption: coeliac disease, tropical sprue, protein energy malnutrition, gastrointestinal infection
  (ii) Haemolytic anaemias: spherocytosis, sickle cell, thalassaemia
  (iii) Artificial diets, goat's milk
  (iv) Drugs: anticonvulsants, antimetabolites, antituberculous, pyrimethamine
3. B_{12}: juvenile pernicious anaemia — vegans, blind loop syndrome, terminal ileum resection
4. Vitamin C: scurvy
5. Rare: vitamin E, cystic fibrosis

Causes of hypoplastic anaemias
1. Aplastic crises: sickle cell, thalassaemia, spherocytosis
2. Metabolic: chronic renal failure, hypothyroidism
3. Drugs, chemicals, radiation
4. Splenomegaly
5. Infiltration: leukaemia, neuroblastoma, tuberculosis
6. Sideroblastic anaemia: X linked pyridoxine responsive, lead poisoning
7. Congenital
  (i) Pure red cell aplasia of Blackfan and Diamond
  (ii) Fanconi's familial pancytopenia with skeletal defects
  (iii) Osteopetrosis

CAUSES OF PURPURA AND BLEEDING: VASCULAR, THROMBOCYTOPENIA, DISORDERED PLATELET FUNCTION, COAGULATION DEFICIENCY

Vascular
1. Trauma
2. Henoch-Schönlein (anaphylactoid) purpura
3. Infection
  (i) Bacterial e.g. meningococcaemia, SBE, septicaemia, scarlet fever, typhoid, Rickettsia, anthrax
  (ii) Viral e.g. measles, infectious mononucleosis, cytomegalovirus
4. Drugs e.g. salicylates, barbiturates, penicillin, sulphonamides
5. Metabolic: scurvy, uraemia
6. Rare
  (i) Inherited: hereditary haemorrhagic telangiectasia, osteogenesis imperfecta, Ehlers-Danlos syndrome, Marfan's syndrome
  (ii) Systemic lupus erythematosus (SLE)

Thrombocytopenia < 150,000/mm³
1. Increased destruction or trapping
   (i) Idiopathic thrombocytopenic purpura: auto-immune, viral
   (ii) Hypersplenism e.g portal hypertension (p. 129), thalassaemia, Gaucher's, etc
   (iii) Infection
       a. Viral: rubella, mumps, measles, chickenpox, cytomegalovirus, infectious mononucleosis
       b. Toxoplasmosis
   (iv) Immunological drug reaction e.g. Sedormid, quinine, sulphas, thiazides, rifampicin
   (v) Consumption
       a. Infectious e.g. meningococcal septicaemia, SBE, etc
       b. Shock: haemorrhagic shock encephalopathy syndrome
       c. Haemolytic uraemic syndrome
       d. Giant haemangioma (Kasabach-Merritt syndrome)
   (vi) Rare: SLE, auto-immune haemolytic anaemia with ITP (Evan's syndrome)
2. Decreased production
   (i) Leukaemia, neuroblastoma, lymphoma
   (ii) Uraemia
   (iii) Hypoplastic anaemias (p. 129)
   (iv) Drugs: chloramphenicol, thiazides, phenylbutazone, etc
   (v) Megaloblastic anaemia

Platelet dysfunction
1. Drugs: aspirin, Dextran infusion
2. Metabolic: uraemia, liver disease
3. Scurvy
4. Inherited
   (i) von Willebrand's disease
   (ii) Thrombasthenia (Glanzmann's disease)
   (iii) Giant platelets (Bernard-Soulier syndrome)

Coagulation deficiency
1. Acquired, increased consumption
   (i) Disseminated intravascular coagulation e.g. shock, asphyxia, sepsis
   (ii) Necrotising enterocolitis
   (iii) Purpura fulminans

2. Acquired, decreased production
    (i) Vitamin K dependent factors: prothrombin VII, IX, X
       a. Haemorrhagic disease of the newborn
       b. Altered bowel flora e.g. infection, antibiotics
       c. Malabsorption
       d. Liver disease
       e. Maternal coumarin medication
3. Inherited
    (i) Haemophilia (factor VIII)
    (ii) Christmas disease (factor IX)
    (iii) von Willebrand's disease (factor VIII, and VIII antigen
       renamed the von Willebrand factor)
    (iv) Others, rare

Immunology

NORMAL DEVELOPMENT OF IMMUNE SYSTEM

1. Fetal: immunoglobulins of G class pass from mother to baby, and are responsible not only for protecting baby but also cause disease e.g. rhesus incompatability, thyrotoxicosis, immune thrombocytopenia, systemic lupus erythematosus
2. Newborn: maternal origin and levels of immunoglobulin G, (IgA and IgM low), falling progressively to very low level by 3 months.

   Neutrophils are active but not yet good at fighting and thus babies are at increased risk of bacterial infection.

   Lymphocyte function (B and T cell) not well developed, manifest by frequent superficial fungal (candida) infection and greater susceptibility to herpes simplex virus.

   Thymus is large and easily seen on X-ray (p. 86). It shrinks rapidly in stress or cyanotic congenital heart disease
3. Infant: breast-feeding protects via IgA, lactoferrin, interferon, lysozyme, maternal macrophages in the milk. Progressive rise in production of own immunoglobulins and cellular immunity

IMMUNE RESPONSE TO MICRO-ORGANISMS

Selected primary immuno-deficiencies

Humoral (B cell)	Pyogenic bacteria, giardia	Gammaglobulin treatment
1. Hypogammaglobulinaemia = total < 2.5 g/l, IgG < 2.0 g/l		
Transient, of infancy	Onset at 4–6 months of age, up to 2 years	
Infantile X linked (Bruton's)	Onset after 6 months old, absent tonsils and lymph glands; malabsorption and arthritis common; no antibodies detected	
2. Selective deficiency		
Isolated IgA (< 50 mg/l)	Mainly respiratory, occasional coeliac; $\frac{1}{3}$ symptomless	
Isolated IgM (< 59 mg/l)	Septicaemia	

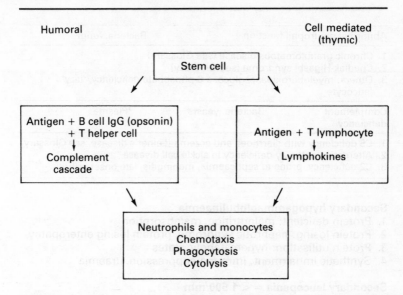

Fig. 23

Thymus (T cell)	Bacteria, viruses, pneumocystitis, fungi

1. Di George: thymus and parathyroid hypoplasia, defects of heart and face, hypocalcaemic fits after day 3, absent thymus on X-ray, severe persistent infections from 3 months: do fetal thymus transplant
2. Chronic mucocutaneous candidiasis ± endocrinopathy: persistent candida infection of mouth, skin, nails: give transfer factor

Stem (B+T cell)	Bacteria, viruses, giardia, candida	Treatment: bone marrow in 1

1. Severe combined immuno-deficiency (SCID): onset after neonatal period. Candida, chronic diarrhoea with persistence of viruses and bacteria. BCG and live vaccine often fatal
   (i) X linked
   (ii) Autosomal recessive: adenosine deaminase deficiency etc
2. Multiple system abnormality: ataxia telangiectasia, Wiskott-Aldrich syndrome, short limb dwarfism with cartilage-hair hypoplasia

Neutropenia	Bacteria	?Bone marrow

1. Autosomal recessive neonatal neutropenia: often fatal
2. Cyclical neutropenia: infections of skin, mouth ulcers, every few weeks
3. With pancreatic insufficiency, normal sweat test: Shwachman syndrome

Abnormal neutrophil function	Bacteria, fungi

1. Chronic granulomatous disease (see Glossary)
2. Chediak-Higashi syndrome (see Glossary)
3. Others: myeloperoxidase, glucose-6-phosphate deficiency, 'lazy', leucocyte

Complement deficiency	Bacteria, yeasts	?Plasma

1. C5 deficiency with diarrhoea and eczema (Leiner's disease, see Glossary)
2. Alternative pathway deficiency in sickle cell disease
3. C2 deficiency, prone to septicaemia, meningitis, late onset arthritis

Secondary hypogammaglobulinaemia
1. Protein deficient: malnutrition, malabsorption
2. Protein losing: nephrotic syndrome, protein losing enteropathy
3. Protein utilisation: hypercatabolic states
4. Synthetic impairment: immuno-suppression, uraemia

Secondary leucopenia = < 1 500/mm
1. Infection: septicaemia, typhoid, brucellosis, Rickettsia, infectious mononucleosis, influenza, measles, malaria, mycoplasma, AIDS, etc
2. Drugs
   (i) Maternal drugs (e.g. thiazides, phenytoin) or antibodies in the newborn
   (ii) Chloramphenicol etc
3. Hypoplastic anaemias (p. 129)
4. Megaloblastic anaemia

CAUSES OF RECURRENT INFECTION
1. Normal development of immunity
2. Socio-economic, and infants who are bottle-fed (hygiene) or whose parents smoke
3. Secondary to disease:
   (i) Malnutrition
   (ii) Steroids, other drugs i.e. side-effect of treatment
   (iii) Underlying disorder e.g. cystic fibrosis, sickle cell
   (iv) Structural abnormality e.g. cleft palate and otitis media
4. Primary and acquired immune-deficiency of immunoblobulins, white cells or complement systems

Allergy

A state of altered reactivity, i.e. a change in the host's response after exposure to a 'foreign' (allergenic) substance, e.g. drugs, environmental or host's body constituents

Type and clinical onset	Reaction	Examples
I. Anaphylactic or reagin-dependent Onset: immediate	Reaginic *antibody (IgE) bound to tissue cells* (e.g. mast cells) on contact with an antigen (e.g. pollen) → release of histamine, bradykinin, etc	(i) Anaphylaxia (ii) Hay fever, asthma (iii) Urticaria (iv) Food allergies (v) Drug allergies
II: Cytotoxic Onset: minutes to hours	Circulating antibody (IgG or IgM) reacts with *antigen bound to cell* surface, usually in presence of complement → cell damage	(i) Post-streptococcal glomerulonephritis (ii) Rhesus, ABO iso-immunisation (iii) Blood transfusion reactions
III: Circulating immune complexes, the Arthus phenomemon Onset: hours to days	*Freely circulating* antigen and antibody combine in presence of complement to form microprecipitates, and damage to small blood vessels	(i) Henoch-Schönlein purpura (ii) Serum sickness (iii) Allergic pulmonary interstitial alveolitis
IV: Cell mediated, or delayed hyper-sensitivity Onset: days	Sensitised lymphocytes react with an antigen deposited at a local site and release lymphokines such as mitogenic factor (lymphocytes proliferate) and migration inhibition factor (lymphocytes remain stationary)	(i) Eczema (ii) Contact dermatitis (iii) Tuberculin tests

An alternative pragmatic classification. From Warner 1985, by permission of the author and the publisher.

Timing of the reaction after antigen exposure	Nosology	Reaction patterns
Immediate	Cause obvious, except when due to azo dyes and/or preservatives	Anaphylaxis Angio-oedema Urticaria
Immediate and/or late	Cause established only by controlled challenge as natural exposure prolonged or repeated	Vomiting/Diarrhoea Failure to thrive Eczema Rhinitis Asthma
	Mechanism of association with food intolerance controversial	Infantile colic Migraine ± epilepsy
Not established	No established association with food intolerance	Hyperactivity Sudden infant death syndrome
Non-existent	Requires careful assessment by psychiatrist and 'allergist'	Allergy by proxy or the allergic form of Munchausen's syndrome

RECOMMENDED READING

Soothill J F, Hayward A R, Wood C B S 1983 Paediatric immunology Blackwell, Oxford

Warner J O 1985 Allergies in Childhood. In: Macfarlane J A (ed) Progress in child health. Vol 2. Churchill Livingstone, Edinburgh pp 63–76

Oncology

Incidence of malignancy one in 600 in childhood, third commonest cause of death. (Commonest: accidents, then infection)

RELATIVE FREQUENCIES OF COMMON MALIGNANCIES

1. Leukaemia: acute lymphoblastic in 80%
2. Lymphoma
3. Cerebral tumours: astrocytoma, medulloblastoma. Seventy per cent are infratentorial
4. Neuroblastoma
5. Wilms' tumour
6. Bone: Ewing's tumour, osteogenic sarcoma

COMMON AGE AT PRESENTATION OF MALIGNANCIES

2–4 years: Acute lymphoblastic leukaemia (ALL)
            Wilm's tumour of kidney
            Neuroblastoma
7 years: Lymphoma (non-Hodgkin's)
            Ewing's sarcoma of bone
≥10 years: Acute myeloid leukaemia

LEUKAEMIA

Characteristics of 'good risk' for ALL:
Aged 1–10 years, Caucasian, girl, anaemic, low WBC (< 5000) platelets plentiful, no significant lympadenopathy or mediastinal widening on X-ray (plus 'null' cell, i.e. non-T, non-B cell markers in the bone marrow, which returns to normal within 14 days of optimal treatment)

Characteristics of 'bad risk' for ALL:
Infant or adolescent, boy, Black, normal Hb, very high WBC, low platelets, diffuse lymphadenopathy and mediastinal glands, T cell bone marrow cell markers and incomplete response to treatment by bone marrow or CSF containing leukaemic cells

137

CAUSES OF HIGH WBC with excessively elevated lymphocytes

1. Glandular fever, cytomegalovirus (both have atypical lymphocytes)
2. Pertussis (cough is obvious)
3. Still's disease (p. 102) (may be difficult to differentiate clinically from leukaemia)
4. Leukaemia

CHARACTERISTICS OF CEREBRAL TUMOURS

Most (70%) are infratentorial in the posterior fossa and symptoms are those of:
1. Raised intracranial pressure e.g. headache ± vomiting
2. Ataxia due to cerebellar involvement. May be unilateral or bilateral depending on site of tumour
3. Cranial nerve palsies due to infiltration and a false localising signs from raised intracranial pressure (VIth cranial nerve)
4. Torticollis

DIFFERENTIAL DIAGNOSIS OF WILMS' TUMOUR, ABDOMINAL NEUROBLASTOMA AND HYDRONEPHROSIS

	Wilms'	Neuroblastoma	Hydronephrosis
Age in years	<5	<5	Any
Health	Well	Usually ill, lethargic	Well
Clinical	Swollen abdomen	Pale, weight loss, diffuse bone pain common	Swollen abdomen, localised pain likely
Mass	Lobulated, firm	Irregular edge, 'craggy', hard	Smooth, tense
Crosses midline	Rare	Common	No
Bilateral	Rare	Occasional	Quite common
IVP pelvis	Grossly distorted	Pushed down, by mass above	Distended, may not work i.e. no dye
Metastases	Lungs	Bone (orbits classically)	

RADIOLOGICAL FEATURES OF MALIGNANCY

1. Vertebral collapse may result from metastatic deposits, but intervertebral disc space preserved. In pyogenic infection both are affected

2. Metaphyseal involvement in neuroblastoma, leukaemia, as well as infections, vitamin deficiencies and lead poisoning is a consequence of its great metabolic activity. Hence always look at ends of long bones carefully
3. (i) Malignant tumour: poorly defined edges, periosteal reaction, destruction of structure, often painful with soft tissue swelling
   (ii) Benign tumour/cyst: well defined border, bone swelling, no bone destruction or periosteal reaction, usually pain free

SIDE EFFECTS OF TREATMENT BY DRUGS AND RADIATION

Common
1. General: nausea, vomiting, fever and diarrhoea
2. Immuno-suppression
3. Bone marrow depression
4. Alopecia
5. Stomatitis, proctitis
6. Skeletal and soft tissue growth impairment

Specific toxicities
1. Cushingoid: prednisolone
2. Hepatotoxicity: cytosine arabinoside, methotrexate, CCNU, asparaginase
3. Neurological
   (i) Encephalopathy : methotrexate
   (ii) Depression: procarbazine
   (iii) Acute ataxia: 5-fluorouracil
   (iv) Neuromuscular weakness: vincristine
4. Lung
   (i) Pulmonary fibrosis: busulphan, bleomycin
   (ii) Pneumonitis: methotrexate
5. Cardiotoxicity: adriamycin, daunorubicin
6. Haemorrhagic cystitis: cyclophosphamide
7. Abdominal pain, constipation: vincristine, vinblastine
8. Dermatitis, hyper-pigmentation: bleomycin, busulphan, cyclophosphamide
9. Infertility: cyclophosphamide, chlorambucil
10. Miscellaneous: malignancy, mental dullness

Renal disorders

NORMAL FINDINGS IN INFANCY

1. Neonatal abdominal palpation: thumb anteriorly, the fingers supporting the back, while the other hand flexes the legs, enabling size and shape of retroperitoneal structures to be assessed. The kidneys move headwards in expiration
2. Boys
   (i) Prepuce retractible in 90% by 4 years old; rare not to retract by puberty
   (ii) Testes undescended in 3% of infants born at term, 1% at 1 year (more frequent in prematures). If absent bilaterally consider intersex (p. 39). Maldescended testes go ectopic, to superficial inguinal pouch, femoral, perineal or pubic areas. Undescended testes follow the normal line of descent
   (iii) Hydrocoeles usually communicate with abdomen, disappear by 1 year and transluminate always, though hernias often do too. Fingers get above former, not hernias
   (iv) Hypoplastic looking penis may be normal but 'buried' in fat pad, as a variation on normal, or small due to hypopituitarism, gonadal dysgenesis or Prader-Willi syndrome
3. Girls
   (i) Some enlargement of the clitoris is normal in the newborn. If excessive, consider virilisation (p. 39), especially congenital adrenal hyperplasia (p. 50)
   (ii) Adhesion of the labia minora. Absent at birth, it appears as an almost transparent line of fusion between the labia, from behind, forwards. Cause unknown; responds to oestrogen cream; tends to recur
   (iii) Prepubertal vaginal mucosa is pink. Oestrogens turn it a velvety-red
4. Renal function
   (i) Glomerular filtration rate is disproportionately low and proportional to gestational age, rising to adult values by 9 months

(ii) Ability to concentrate urine to 600 mOsmol/kg water within the first few months of life. Adult values, up to 1500 mOsmol/kg, after 6 months
(iii) Acidification of urine is limited and renal bicarbonate threshold low at 21 mmol/l (adult 25 mmol/l). Infants are therefore more easily made acidaemic
(iv) Phosphate excretion limited in neonate, with hypoparathyroidism from relative maternal hyperparathyroidism. Hypocalcaemia is likely when fed unmodified cow's milk
(v) For the first 2 weeks of extrauterine life a preterm infant of less than 32 weeks' gestation has a reduced ability to resorb sodium; enhanced reabsorption of creatinine is reflected in higher serum values

RENAL DISORDERS BY AGE AT PRESENTATION

Neonate and infant
1. Urinary tract infection (males > females)
   (i) Haematogenous
   (ii) Ascending, obstructive (p. 145)
   (iii) Fistulous e.g. rectal atresia (boys)
2. Renal failure (p. 147) e.g. Potter's renal agenesis syndrome, dysplasia, obstructive lesions, congenital nephrosis
3. Nephrogenic diabetes insipidus

Toddlers and older
1. Urinary tract infection (females > males). Ascending infection common, obstructive and haematogenous less so
2. Minimal change nephrotic syndrome
3. Haemolytic uraemic syndrome
4. Congenital disorders: cystinosis, renal tubular acidosis

Childhood
1. Overt urinary tract infection and 'asymptomatic' bacteriuria (females > males)
2. Acute and chronic glomerulonephritis
3. Familial nephritis

SOME CAUSES OF COLOURED URINE AND NAPPIES

Urine
1. Dark yellow: concentrated, bile
2. Pink to dark red
   (i) Blood, haemoglobinuria, myoglobinuria
   (ii) Drugs and dyes e.g. phenolphthalein, senna, beeturia
   (iii) Porphyria, congenital erythropoietic

3. Black
    (i) Alcaptonuria, tyrosinosis, melaninuria
    (ii) Drugs e.g. methyl dopa

Nappy
1. Red
    (i) Urates (in concentrated urine — may be mistaken for haematuria, especially in boys
    (ii) Serratia marcescens (in napkin soiled for 24 hours)
2. Blue
    (i) Hypercalcaemia (in blue diaper syndrome)
    (ii) Pseudomonas aeruginosa in towel napkin
3. Orange sand: Lesch-Nyhan syndrome

CAUSES OF A POSITIVE BENEDICT'S (CLINITEST) REACTION

1. Clinistix positive: glycosuria e.g. diabetes mellitus (p. 48)
2. Clinistix negative
    (i) Galactosaemia
    (ii) Hereditary fructosaemia
    (iii) Benign fructosuria, pentosuria, lactosuria
    (iv) Alcaptonuria (black)
    (v) Vitamin C, other drugs

CAUSES OF KETONURIA (POSITIVE ACETEST OR KETOSTIX)

1. Starvation, persistent vomiting
2. Acute febrile illness
3. Diabetes mellitus
4. Ketotic hypoglycaemia
5. Inborn errors e.g. glycogenoses, I, III (p. 152), organic acidurias, lactic acidosis

CAUSES OF FREQUENCY OF MICTURITION

1. Physiological age related, stress, cold weather
2. Emotional: attention seeking
3. Urinary tract abnormality
    (i) Infection
    (ii) Ureteric reflux (gross)
    (iii) Obstruction e.g. neurogenic bladder, posterior urethral valves
4. Metabolic: diabetes mellitus, diabetes insipidus, hypercalcaemia, renal failure, renal tubular acidosis
5. Pelvic appendicitis
6. Antihistamine
7. Calculi

CAUSES OF OLIGURIA OR ANURIA

1. Retention of urine
   - (i) Neurogenic: poliomyelitis, polyneuritis, coma etc
   - (ii) Local inflammation e.g. vulvo-vaginitis, meatal ulcer
   - (iii) Emotional
2. Dehydration
3. Shock
4. Acute glomerulonephritis
5. Nephrotic syndrome
6. Chronic renal failure
7. Miscellaneous: acute tubular necrosis, bilateral cortical necrosis, renal vein thrombosis, haemolytic uraemic syndrome
8. Side-effects
   - (i) Transfusion reaction
   - (ii) Crystaluria: sulphonamides, antileukaemic therapy

Differentiation of pre-renal from renal failure

	Pre-renal	Renal
1. Urine: plasma creatinine ratio of > 5.0	↑	↓
2. Urine: plasma osmolality ratio of > 1.3	↑	↓

CAUSES OF POLYURIA

1. Polydipsia: psychogenic, attention seeking
2. Urinary tract infection
3. Diabetes mellitus
4. Diabetes insipidus
5. Miscellaneous renal: chronic renal failure, acute tubular necrosis, renal tubular acidosis, Fanconi's syndrome (p. 146)
6. Metabolic: hypercalcaemia, hypokalaemic nephropathy, Conn's primary hyperaldosteronism
7. Sickle cell disease

CAUSES OF ENURESIS

1. Primary: physiological, emotional, mental retardation
2. Onset enuresis
   - (i) Emotional
   - (ii) Urinary tract infection
   - (iii) Diabetes mellitus, diabetes insipidus
   - (iv) Obstruction with overflow
   - (v) Neurogenic bladder
   - (vi) Epilepsy
   - (vii) Sexual abuse

CAUSES OF HAEMATURIA

1. Trauma
2. Infection
   - (i) Acute bacterial urinary tract infection
   - (ii) Leptospirosis, syphilis, schistosomiasis, tuberculosis
   - (iii) Bacterial endocarditis, infected ventriculo-atrial shunt
   - (iv) Viral: infectious mononucleosis, acute haemorrhagic cystitis (adenovirus)
3. Acute glomerulonephritis
4. Henoch-Schönlein (anaphylactoid) purpura
5. Benign recurrent haematuria: fever, exercise, familial, Berger's disease
6. Chronic glomerulonephritis
7. Munchausen by proxy
8. Calculi
9. Haematological
   - (i) Bleeding: haemophilia, thrombocytopenia
   - (ii) Sickle cell anaemia
10. Tumour: nephroblastoma, rhabdomyosarcoma of bladder
11. Rare: haemoglobinuria, renal haemangioma, systemic lupus erythematosus, Goodpasture's syndrome, polyarteritis nodosa, familial nephritis with deafness (Alport's syndrome)

SOME CAUSES OF PYURIA

Common

1. Physiological: girls, bag urine, not spun, 50–100/mm^3, otherwise clean voided < 10/mm^3
2. Urinary tract infection
3. Dehydration, fever
4. Genital infection e.g. vulvo-vaginitis, balanitis, urethritis
5. Trauma
6. Drugs e.g. cyclophosphamide

Unusual

1. Renal tubular acidosis, nephrocalcinosis, calculi, renal TB
2. Kawasaki disease

CAUSES OF FLANK MASSES

1. Unilateral
   (i) Multicystic kidney
   (ii) Solitary or multiple kidney cysts
   (iii) Hydronephrosis
   (iv) Trauma
   (v) Tumour e.g. Wilms'
2. Bilateral
   (i) Hydronephrosis
      a. Outlet obstruction e.g. posterior urethral valves,
         ureterocoeles, urethral stricture, foreign body, stone,
         faecal impaction
      b. Neurogenic bladder e.g. spina bifida, diastematomyelia,
         sacral agenesis, transverse myelitis
      c. Megacystis: diabetes insipidus, prune belly syndrome
   (ii) Cystic disease
      a. Infantile autosomal recessive polycystic disease
      b. Adult autosomal dominant polycystic disease
      c. Lowe's occulo-cerebro-renal syndrome
      d. Tuberous sclerosis
   (iii) Tumour: Wilms', leukaemia, lymphoma
   (iv) Renal vein thrombosis

CAUSES OF NEPHROTIC SYNDROME (proteinuria > 3 g/day)

1. Minimal change
2. Secondary
   (i) Henoch-Schönlein (anaphylactoid) purpura
   (ii) Post nephritic
   (iii) Membranous
   (iv) Membranoproliferative
   (v) Quartan malaria nephrosis — common in endemic areas
   (vi) Renal vein thrombosis
   (vii) Toxins: troxidone, lead, mercury, snake bite
   (viii) Allergic: bee sting, pollen, immunisation
   (ix) Miscellaneous: amyloid, sickle cell disease, lupus
        erythematosus
3. Congenital

COMMON FEATURES OF ACUTE NEPHRITIS AND NEPHROTIC SYNDROME

	Nephritis	Nephrosis
Cause	Group Aβ H. streptococcus; Henoch Schönlein; idiopathic	Unknown in 90%
Age	5–15 years, rarely pre-school	Mainly pre-school, up to 10 years
Onset	Sudden	Days or weeks
Mode	Haematuria	Oedema
Temperature	Elevated	Normal
BP	May be raised	Normal*
Urine { protein	++/+++	++++ (Albustix)
blood	++/+++	Absent*
casts	Red cell	Hyaline/fatty
Plasma protein	Normal	Low albumin
Cholesterol	Normal	Raised
ASOT	Raised	Normal
C3 complement	Low	Normal
Prognosis	Good in 95%	Good unless raised blood urea/*BP, *haematuria; age < 1 or > 10 years

ASOT = Antistreptolysin O titre
BP = blood pressure

CAUSES OF RENAL TUBULAR ACIDOSIS

Proximal
1. Renal Fanconi syndrome (damage causing leak of bicarbonate, phosphate, glucose, amino acid, protein, potassium)
    (i) Inherited e.g. cystinosis, galactosaemia, Wilson's disease, tyrosinaemia, hereditary fructose intolerance, Lowe's occulo-cerebral-renal syndrome
   (ii) Nephrotic syndrome
  (iii) Hyperparathyroidism
  (iv) Toxins
        a. Metals, e.g. lead, cadmium, mercury
        b. Lysol, outdated tetracycline, neomycin
2. Primary renal tubular acidosis: bicarbonate reabsoprtion alone is affected

Distal (impaired hydrogen ion excretion, urine pH 6.0 or more)
1. Lightwood's transient renal tubular acidosis
2. Permanent renal tubular acidosis
    (i) Familial
   (ii) Phenacetin, amphotericin B

3. Miscellaneous
   (i) Renal tubular necrosis
   (ii) Chronic renal failure

CAUSES OF ACUTE RENAL FAILURE

1. Pre-renal
   (i) Dehydration
   (ii) Shock: septicaemia, operations, burns, Reye's syndrome
   (iii) Cardiac failure
   (iv) Nephrotic syndrome
   (v) Renal vein thrombosis
2. Renal
   (i) Acute glomerulonephritis
   (ii) Trauma
   (iii) Urinary tract infection
   (iv) Toxins e.g. ethylene glycol, CCl_4, mercury
   (v) Drugs e.g. frusemide, cephalosporins, gentamycin, sulphas, phenytoin
   (vi) Miscellaneous: haemolytic uraemic syndrome, burns, dysplastic kidneys
3. Post-renal
   (i) Obstruction
      a. Posterior urethral valves, clots
      b. Ureteric obstruction of a single kidney
   (ii) Crystals: sulphonamides, uric acid in antileukaemic therapy

COMMONER CAUSES OF ACUTE RENAL FAILURE BY AGE

Infants
1. Pre-renal: acute gastroenteritis, septicaemia, congenital heart disease, renal vein thrombosis
2. Renal: urinary tract infection, haemolytic uraemic syndrome
3. Post-renal: posterior urethral valves

Children
1. Pre-renal: acute dehydration, trauma, burns, scalds, nephrotic syndrome
2. Renal: acute glomerulonephritis, acute tubular necrosis due to pre-renal cause
3. Post-renal: neurogenic e.g. acute myelitis, cord compression

CAUSES OF CHRONIC RENAL FAILURE

1. Glomerulonephritis
2. Pyelonephritis
3. Hydronephrosis, obstructive uropathy } See causes of flank
4. Renal hypoplasia, dysplasia   } masses (p. 145)

5. Cortical or tubular necrosis
6. Miscellaneous: Henoch-Schönlein (anaphylactoid) purpura, haemolytic uraemic syndrome
7. Cystic disease
8. Hereditary
    (i) Nephritis e.g. Alport's syndrome (p. 144)
    (ii) Metabolic: cystinosis, Wilson's disease

CAUSES OF DETERIORATION IN RENAL FUNCTION IN CHRONIC RENAL FAILURE

1. Primary disease
2. Infection
3. Hypertension
4. Drug nephrotoxicity
5. Biochemical
    (i) Salt depletion
    (ii) Hypercalcaemia
    (iii) Phosphate retention
    (iv) Protein toxicity (hyperfiltration)
6. Obstruction

FURTHER READING

Anderson G F, Smey P 1985 Current concepts in the management of common urological problems in infants and children. Pediatric Clinics of North America. Vol. 32 (5). Saunders, Philadelphia, pp. 1133–1149
Gauthier B, Edelman C M, Barnett H L 1982 Nephrology and urology for the pediatrician. Little, Brown, Boston

Metabolic disorders

ACID-BASE DISORDERS

Infants have lower plasma bicarbonate (18–24 mmol/l) than older children and adults, because the renal threshold is lower. They are therefore less able to acidify their urine and have less reserve (or defence) against acidosis

Characteristics of acid-base disorders:

	pH	pCO$_2$	Base Excess	Std. HCO$_3$
Metabolic acidosis	Down	Down*	− n	Down
Metabolic alkalosis	Up	Up*	+ n	Up
Respiratory acidosis	Down	Up	+ n	Up*
Respiratory alkalosis	Up	Down	− n	Down*

* After allowing time for compensation: quick respiratory = pCO$_2$ (mins) slow metabolic = standard HCO$_3$ (hours)
n = number of mmol/l of acid (−) or alkali (+) to be corrected to achieve 'neutrality'
Correction of negative base excess (base deficit)
= body weight (kg) × base deficit × 0.3
= number of mmol alkaline (sodium bicarbonate) need

METABOLIC ACIDOSIS (low pH, low total CO$_2$ content)

1. Loss of bicarbonate
   (i) Bowel: diarrhoea, fistula
   (ii) Renal: renal tubular acidosis, Fanconi's syndrome (p. 146)
2. Gain of strong acid
   (i) Lactic acid e.g. respiratory distress syndrome (RDS), anoxia, septicaemia, shock, leukaemia, glycogen storage disease
   (ii) Keto-acids e.g. starvation, diabetes mellitus
   (iii) Ingestion e.g. salicylates, chlorides of ammonia and calcium
   (iv) Dietary sulphuric acid in sulphated amino acids e.g. acidosis of prematurity, chronic renal failure
   (v) Various organic acids and amino acid ketones in inborn errors of metabolism e.g. maple syrup urine disease, proprionic acidaemia

3. Miscellaneous
    (i) Saline infusion (pH 7.0) in excess (by dilution)
    (ii) Carbonic acid anhydrase inhibitor

METABOLIC ALKALOSIS (high pH, high total CO_2 content)

Intracellular acidosis may occur e.g. in hypokalaemia, when paradoxical acid urine may be found
1. Loss of acid
    (i) Vomiting e.g. pyloric stenosis
    (ii) Diuretics
    (iii) Cushing's, Conn's syndrome
    (iv) Hypokalaemia: commonly (i), (ii), (iii) and chronic renal disease (p. 147), malabsorption (H^+ shifts intracellularly to replace K^+ loss)
2. Gain of alkali: excessive ingestion

RESPIRATORY ALKALOSIS (high pH, low total CO_2 content)

1. Physiological: hysteria, fever
2. Central: encephalitis, trauma, tumour, early salicylate poisoning
3. Peripheral, i.e. compensatory mechanism, in e.g. hypoxia, metabolic acidosis, pneumonitis, pulmonary oedema

RESPIRATORY ACIDOSIS (low pH, high total CO_2 content)

1. Central: sedatives, head injury, encephalitis, polyneuritis
2. Obstruction of airways e.g. foreign body, epiglottitis, asthma
3. Parenchymal, e.g. respiratory distress syndrome (RDS), acute pneumonia, pneumothorax, chronic scoliosis, cystic fibrosis
4. Assisted ventilation: rate too low, volume too small, wrong inspiratory: expiratory ratio, disconnection, large dead space etc

MIXED DISORDERS

Examples
1. Respiratory alkalosis, metabolic acidosis in salicylate poisoning
2. Respiratory acidosis, metabolic acidosis in RDS, cystic fibrosis, shock, hypothermia

CAUSES OF HYPOCALCAEMIA

Newborn (p. 23)   < 1.8 mmol/
Infancy   < 2.1 mmol/
1. Rickets
    (i) Lack of normal requirements: sun, vitamin D, calcium; excess of phytates (e.g. in chapatis)
    (ii) Anticonvulsants: increased vitamin D turnover
    (iii) Increased normal requirements: premature
    (iv) Malabsorption e.g. coeliac disease

  (v) Hepatic e.g. cirrhosis, biliary obstruction
  (iv) Renal: chronic renal failure
2. Alkalosis
   (i) Pyloric stenosis
   (ii) Hyperventilation
   (iii) Excess alkali intake
3. Renal rickets
   (i) Vitamin D dependent
   (ii) Hypophosphataemic rickets: familial vitamin D resistant,
         renal tubular acidosis, generalised tubular disorder e.g.
         Fanconi's
4. Addison's disease
5. Hypomagnesaemia, primary and secondary to steatorrhoea
6. Hypoparathyroidism

Biochemical differentiation of types of hypoparathyroidism

	Comment
Idiopathic	Low calcium low parathormone (PTH) = deficient in PTH
Pseudo-	Low calcium, normal PTH = resistant to PTH
Pseudo-pseudo-	Normal biochemistry = a phenocopy

CAUSES OF HYPERCALCAEMIA

1. Infancy
   (i) Idiopathic hypercalcaemia of infancy (part of William's
        syndrome)
   (ii) Vitamin D intoxication
   (iii) Subcutaneous fat necrosis (birth trauma)
2. Any age
   (i) Steroid withdrawal
   (ii) Malignancy with bone deposits
   (iii) Immobilisation
   (iv) Endocrine
        a. Hyperparathyroidism: primary, tertiary
        b. Thyrotoxicosis
        c. Multiple endocrine neoplasia
   (v) Hypophosphatasia

Biochemical differentiation of hypercalcaemia in infancy

Disorder	Blood concentration of:		
	Parathormone	Phosphate	Vitamin D
Hyperparathyroidism	↑	↓	Normal
Hypervitaminosis D	Normal	Normal	↑
Idiopathic hypercalcaemia	Normal	Normal	Normal

CARBOHYDRATE DISORDERS

Rare, autosomal recessive inheritance
1. Glycogen storage disorders
   Enzyme deficiency of glycogen metabolism in liver and/or muscle
   (i) Primary hepatic: types I, III, IV, VI
       Type I (von Gierke's): infantile onset of failure to thrive, enlarged liver and kidneys. Hypoglycaemia with ketosis, elevated blood lactic acid, uric acid and triglycerides. Platelet defect. Death aged 1–40 years old
       Type IV (Amylopectinosis): onset of progressive cirrhosis in infancy. Death by 2 years
       Other types: mild growth failure, hepatomegaly, asymptomatic hypoglycaemia, easily fatigued
   (ii) Myopathic: types II, V, VII, VIII
       Type II (Pompe's): infantile variety, hypotonia, enlarged tongue and heart from neonatal period. Heart failure and death by 2 years
       Type V (McArdle's) and others: muscle cramps on exercise with myoglobinuria. Childhood onset
2. Galactosaemia
   Enzyme deficiency: galactose-1-phosphate uridyl transferase
   Onset: as milk feeding is established
   Symptoms: vomiting, apathy, prolonged jaundice, failure to thrive
   Signs: hepatosplenomegaly, cataracts
   Treatment: low lactose, Nutramigen or Galactomin milk

HYPERLIPIDAEMIAS OF PAEDIATRIC IMPORTANCE

1. Primary hyperchylomicronaemia, or Type I autosomal recessive: lipoprotein lipase deficiency. Recurrent abdominal pain ± xanthomata, hepatosplenomegaly, lipaemia retinalis. Fasting serum is turbid (chylomicrons ++), triglycerides +++, cholesterol +; also secondary to poorly controlled diabetes mellitus or von Gierke's disease
2. Familial hypercholesterolaemia, or Type IIa autosomal dominant. Xanthomata, arcus senilis, ischaemic heart disease in childhood in homozygote, early in adult life in heterozygote. Serum cholesterol normal <6.2 mmol/l, heterozygote 7–13 mmol/l, homozygote 20–25 mmol/l. Increased beta-lipoprotein

AMINO ACIDURIAS

Type	Clinical features	1. Enzyme defect 2. Milk (brand)
Phenylketonuria (PKU)	'Mousy' smell, eczema, fair hair, blue eyes, psychomotor slowing, fits, cerebral palsy, autistic behaviour. Onset 3–5 months	1. Phenylalanine hydroxylase and variants 2. Lofenalac, Albumaid XP etc
Maple syrup urine disease* (MSUD)	'Caramel' smell, convulsions, cerebral oedema, hypoglycaemia, ketoacidosis. Onset age 1 week. Death in weeks if untreated	1. Branched chain decarboxylase 2. SMUD Aid
Hereditary tyrosinaemia	Failure to thrive, hepatosplenomegaly, liver failure, renal tubular acidosis. Renal rickets, hypoglycaemia. Onset in infancy	1. p-Hydroxyphenyl pyruvic acid oxidase 2. Albumaid X phenylalanine and tyrosine
Homocystinuria	Mental retardationin 50%, hypertension, Marfan-like stature, lens dislocation	1. Cystathione synthetase or folate 2. Albumaid X methionine, or give pyridoxine (B6), B12
Histidinaemia	? Mild mental retardation	1. Histidase 2. ? Low histidine diet

* Organic acidaemias and urea cycle defects have similar clinical presentation except smell

1. Normal plasma amino acid level
   (i) Proximal tubular damage e.g. Fanconi's syndrome (p. 146), cystinosis)
   (ii) Renal tubular cell transport defect e.g. Hartnup's disease, cystinuria
2. Elevated plasma amino acid levels (PKU commonest, autosomal recessive inheritance)

SPHINGOLIPIDOSES

Lysosomal enzyme deficiency, resulting in excess accumulation of a normally synthesised product
Onset in infancy, excepting Batten's. Death within 1–5 years after onset. Enzyme deficiency identifiable in leucocytes. Autosomal recessive inheritance

Type	Clinical features
Batten's group	Convulsions, progressive dementia and failure of vision. Characteristic EEG and electro-retinogram changes in late infantile and juvenile types of onset
Tay-Sach's	Psychomotor deterioration, tetraplegia, 'hyperacusis', cherry red macula
Gaucher's	Infantile: psychomotor deterioration, tetraplegia, hepatomegaly Chronic: hepatosplenomegaly, hypersplenism, aseptic bone necrosis, normal IQ
Niemann-Pick's	Psychomotor deterioration, blindness, cherry red spot, pulmonary infiltrates, hepatosplenomegaly
Generalised gangliosidosis, GM$_1$	CNS: Tay-Sach's like Somatic: Hurler like

PURINE INHERITED METABOLIC ERRORS

1. Lesch-Nyhan's syndrome
2. Adenosine deaminase deficiency

MUCOPOLYSACCHARIDOSES (Autosomal recessive inheritance except for Hunter's)

Excessive storage and urinary excretion of heparan sulphate and dermatan sulphate. Morquio's excrete keratan sulphate. All are rare
1. Type I Hurler
    (i) Somatic features: grotesque facies, corneal opacities, dwarfism, stiff limbed, skeletal deformities, enlarged tongue, hepatosplenomegaly
    (ii) CNS features: progressive psychomotor retardation
    (iii) Heart: valves become incompetent, causing failure
2. Hurler-like: Type II Hunter — a sex linked condition
                Type VII neonatal onset, severe
3. Somatic changes only:
    Type I Scheie, mildly affected
    Type IV Morquio, severe ligamentous laxity, normal facies, severe kyphosis
    Type VI Maroteaux-Lamy
4. CNS changes mainly:
    Type III Sanfilippo, severe mental retardation

FURTHER READING

Rendle-Short J, Gray O P, Dodge J A 1984 A synopsis of children's diseases. Sections 7 & 8. 6th edn. Wright, Bristol, pp 139–169

Orthopaedics

NORMAL POSTURAL VARIATIONS

Neonate
Intrauterine position commonly causes postural deformities of feet. Limbs assume 'position of comfort'

Infant
Pigeon toe (metatarsus varus) is normal if passively correctable. Curly, overlapping toes usually self correct

Toddler
Flat feet and bow legs to 2 years. Gap between medial femoral condyles up to 10 cm is normal; if more see p. 157

Pre-school
Knock-knees 2 to 6 years, more than 10 cm intermaleolar gap is likely to be pathological (p. 157)

School age
Straight legs are to be expected

Any age
In-toeing (pigeon toe) or out-toeing (Charlie Chaplin Walk) is usually due to normal degrees of tibial torsion, anteversion or retroversion of the neck of the femur, knock knees (p. 157) or bow legs (p. 157)

N.B. 1. Asymmetry is always suspicious: consider congenital abnormality, trauma, or tumour
    2. Symmetrical deformity: endocrine, metabolic disorder is more likely

SCREENING

Congenital dislocation of the hip
1. Neonate: see p. 13
2. Infant: the "classical" signs, commoner after 6 weeks old

   a. One hip: shorter leg, **limited abduction**, extra skin fold, asymmetric buttock folds, 'telescoping' may be elicited (p. 13). If walking, Trendelenburg dip (p. 157) present when taking weight on affected leg

   b. Bilateral: wide perineum, limited abduction, waddling walk

Scoliosis
To exclude a postural curve the erect child should bend forward, arms hanging loosely down. If one shoulder is still higher than the other, repeat forward flexion with child seated to eliminate asymmetry of leg length as the cause

CAUSES OF FLAT FOOT

1. Pes planus: heel symmetrically on the floor
   (i) Racial
   (ii) Ligamentous laxity
2. Pes planovalgus: heel everted, medial border of foot bulging
   (i) Trauma
   (ii) Neurological: cerebral palsy, poliomyelitis, myelomeningocoele
   (iii) Congenital vertical talus

CAUSES OF CLUB FOOT

Talipes equinovarus: foot down, medially rotated
Talipes calcaneovalgus: heel down, foot laterally rotated
1. Intrauterine posture
2. Familial
3. Secondary to spina bifida, poliomyelitis
4. Arthrogryposis
5. Vertical talus, cerebral palsy in equinovarus only
NB: Walking on tip toe is seen in some normal toddlers, in spastic diplegia, congenital shortening of the tendo Achilles, early muscular dystrophy, dystonia musculorum deformans and autism.

CAUSES OF OUT-TOEING (externally rotated foot)

1. Physiological tibial torsion (especially very premature infants laid in prone), knock knee or femoral retroversion
2. Hip problem: congenital dislocation of the hip, slipped femoral epiphysis, coxa vara
3. Knock knee pathology (p. 157): rickets, cerebral palsy, spina bifida

CAUSES OF IN-TOEING (internally rotated foot)

1. Physiological metatarsus varus, tibial torsion, bow leg, femoral anteversion
2. 'Irritable hip'
3. Bow leg pathology: trauma, rickets, Blount's osteochondritis of the medial tibial condyle
4. Ankle: peroneal muscular atrophy, club foot

CAUSES OF KNOCK KNEE (GENU VALGUM)

1. Physiological
2. Trauma
3. Rickets (p. 150)
4. Neurological: cerebral palsy, poliomyelitis, myelomeningocoele
5. Bone cysts, neurofibromatosis

CAUSES OF BOW LEGS (GENU VARUM)

1. Physiological
2. Trauma
3. Rickets (p. 150)
4. Blount's osteochondritis of the medial tibial metaphysis

CAUSES OF TRENDELENBURG DIP

1. Hip joint — unstable: congenital dislocation of the hip, septic arthritis, tuberculosis
2. Neck of femur (normal angle 135° to femoral shaft) — coxa vara = more acute angle: trauma, late in Perthe's disease or slipped femoral epiphysis, rickets, tuberculosis, osteomyelitis, cerebreal palsy, hypothyroidism
3. Weak hip abductors (mainly gluteus medius): muscle disease e.g. Duchênne, limb girdle dystrophies, poliomyelitis

CAUSES OF SCOLIOSIS

1. Primary
   (i) Postural
   (ii) Idiopathic (80% of all scolioses): infantile, adolescent types
2. Secondary
   (i) Bone: hemivertebrae
   (ii) Ligaments: Marfan's syndrome of tall stature, wide arm span, long digits, lens dislocation, aortic rupture, scoliosis. Autosomal dominant inheritance
   (iii) Muscle: muscular dystrophies
   (iv) Neurogenic: spina bifida, poliomyelitis, cerebral palsy, Freidreich's ataxia

CAUSES OF TORTICOLLIS

1. Muscular
    (i) Congenital sternomastoid 'tumour'
    (ii) Trauma
    (iii) Myositis
2. Cervical adenitis
3. Subluxations
    (i) Trauma
    (ii) Infections of pharynx
4. Ocular
    (i) IV nerve palsy, brain stem tumour
    (ii) Nystagmus, spasmus nutans (abnormal head posture and movements with nystagmus in infancy)
5. Central nervous system
    (i) Posterior fossa tumour
    (ii) Phenothiazine poisoning
6. Vertebral anomalies e.g. Klippel-Feil's fusion of cervical vertebrae, Sprengel's congenitally high shoulder, hemivertebrae
7. Psychological: spasmodic torticollis

CAUSES OF ACUTE PAINFUL JOINT OR LIMP

(remember 'growing pains' and cramps are 2 common conditions with characteristic histories, which must be differentiated from the following causes:

1. Trauma
    (i) Severe
    (ii) Mild, may exacerbate slipped femoral epiphysis (see p. 160)
    (iii) Non-accidental injury
2. Irritable hip
3. Infection: osteomyelitis especially *Staphylococcus aureus*, *Haemophilus influenzae*, tuberculosis, viral e.g. mumps, rubella
4. Henoch-Schönlein purpura (p. 102)
5. Osteochondritis e.g. Perthe's disease of the hip
6. Haematological: sickle cell disease, haemophilia, leukaemia
7. Malignancy: neuroblastoma, histiocytosis X, osteogenic sarcoma, osteoid osteoma
8. Rheumatic fever
9. Iatrogenic: drug reaction, aseptic necrosis and fractures from steroids, serum sickness
10. Myositis

CAUSES OF POLYARTHRITIS

1. Infection
   - (i) Pyogenic e.g. staphylococcal, meningococcal, bacterial endocarditis
   - (ii) Viral e.g. rubella, mumps, glandular fever
   - (iii) Post-infective reaction e.g. salmonella, shigella, yersinia
2. Allergic: Henoch-Schönlein purpura, serum sickness
3. Trauma: non-accidental injury
4. Chronic inflammation
   - (i) Rheumatic fever
   - (ii) Rheumatoid arthritis
   - (iii) Ankylosing spondylitis
   - (iv) Systemic lupus erythematosus
   - (v) Crohn's disease
   - (vi) Ulcerative colitis
5. Haematological: sickle cell disease, haemophilia, and Christmas disease
6. Gout
   - (i) Secondary to antileukaemic therapy, renal failure, von Gierke's disease
   - (ii) Lesch-Nyhan syndrome
7. Rare: hypogammaglobulinaemia, familial Mediterranean fever, hypercholesterolaemia II

COMMON CAUSES OF CHRONIC ARTHRITIS (differential diagnosis of Still's disease)

1. Infective: Mycoplasma pneumoniae, brucellosis, tuberculosis
2. Post-infective: salmonella, shigella
3. Juvenile rheumatoid arthritis (JRA) or Still's disease
4. Chronic bowel disease: Crohn's disease, ulcerative colitis

DIFFERENTIAL DIAGNOSIS OF STILL'S DISEASE, RHEUMATIC FEVER AND HENOCH–SCHÖNLEIN (ANAPHYLACTOID) PURPURA: see p. 102

DIFFERENTIAL DIAGNOSIS OF PATHOLOGY IN HIP, WITH PAIN IN HIP OR REFERRED TO KNEE

	Age in years	Clinical, and leg movement resisted	Investigations
'Irritable hip'	3–10	Usually boy, well, internal rotation, abduction, extension	Normal
Septic hip	0–5+	Toxic, any movement pain++, (lies flexed adducted)	Blood culture +ive, X-ray normal at first, white cell count++, aspirate early
Tuberculosis	2–15	Subacute, stiff and very painful	X-ray: hilar glands? Haemoglobin, white cell count, erythrocyte sedimentation rate, Mantoux test, urine for AAFB
Perthe's	5–10	Usually boy, well, abduction	X-ray: loss of trabeculae, flattening of femoral head
Slipped epiphysis	10–15	Fat/very thin, well, internal rotation, abduction, extension	X-ray: capital epiphysis falling back and downward in lateral view

AAFB: acid and alcohol fast bacilli (tuberculosis)

CAUSES OF FRAGMENTATION OF FEMORAL HEAD ON X-RAY

1. Perthe's disease
2. Avascular necrosis
    (i) Trauma
    (ii) Sickle cell disease, haemophilia
3. Pyogenic arthritis, tuberculosis
4. Iatrogenic: steroids in excess
5. Hypothyroidism
6. Mucopolysaccharidosis

Dermatology

TIME-RELATED CHANGES IN COMMON PIGMENTED LESIONS

Naevus flameus (stork mark) Mongolian blue spot	Fade during first year
Strawberry naevus	Rapid growth in first months, involution complete by 5 years
Café-au-lait patches	Appear during infancy, 6 or more of 1.5 cm diameter or more in von Recklinghausen's disease
Pigmented naevi (various types)	Appear throughout childhood, and in crops if multiple
Spider naevi	Found in healthy children, rarely a sign of chronic liver disease

CAUSES OF ECZEMA

1. Seborrhoeic: alone, with intertrigo or candida (napkin psoriasis)
2. Atopic
3. Infection: scabies
4. Contact dermatitis: medication, lotions, detergents, etc
5. Neurodermatitis
6. Rare: phenylketonuria, histiocytosis X, agammaglobulinaemia, Wiskott-Aldrich syndrome, Leiner's hypocomplementaemia, acrodermatitis enteropathica

CAUSES OF VESICULAR ERUPTIONS

1. Infection
   (i) Viral: herpes zoster, herpes simplex, hand-foot-mouth (Coxsackie A)
   (ii) Bacterial: staphylococcal impetigo and scalded skin syndrome, rickettsial pox, mycoplasma, pseudomonas
   (iii) Scabies (especially neonatal)
2. Urticaria
3. Insect bites: papular urticaria

4. Sweating: malaria, pompholyx
5. Atopic eczema
6. Burns, sunburn
7. Drugs: phenobarbitone, sulphas
8. Pityriasis rosea
9. Rare
    (i) Epidermolysis bullosa: simplex, scarring, lethal types
    (ii) Urticaria pigmentosa, acrodermatitis enteropathica, dermatitis herpetiformis, porphyria

CAUSES OF URTICARIA

1. Allergies
    (i) Foods e.g. shellfish, eggs, cow's milk
    (ii) Food preservatives and dyes
    (iii) Contact: animal hair
    (iv) Inhaled: grain, feathers, house dust, moulds
2. Physical agents: sun, heat, cold, water, pressure
3. Infection: worms, sinusitis
4. Drugs: aspirin, penicillin

CAUSES OF CUTANEOUS CANDIDIASIS

1. Prematurity
2. Bottle-feeding
3. Antibiotic therapy
4. Endocrine: diabetes mellitus, idiopathic hypoparathyroidism, chronic mucocutaneous candidiasis
5. Immunological suppression
    (i) Corticosteroids, antimetabolites
    (ii) Leukaemia
6. Primary immune-deficiency: Di George's syndrome, Bruton's etc

CAUSES OF HAIR LOSS

1. Friction — rubbing head on pillow
2. Post-acute physical/psychological stress
3. Habitual pulling/curling (trichotillomania)
4. Traction alopecia: plaiting etc
5. Alopecia areata
6. Ringworm
7. Drugs: valproate, cytotoxics
8. Miscellaneous: iron deficiency, thyroid disorders

CAUSES OF ERYTHEMA NODUSUM

1. Infection
    (i) Bacterial: streptococcal, meningococcaemia, tuberculosis, psittacosis, yersinia
    (ii) Viral: cat-scratch disease, chlamydia
    (iii) Fungal: coccidioidomycosis, histoplasmosis
2. Drugs: sulphonamides, penicillin
3. Miscellaneous: sarcoidosis, ulcerative colitis, Crohn's disease

CAUSES OF ERYTHEMA MULTIFORME

1. Infection
    (i) Viral: herpes simplex, glandular fever, chlamydia
    (ii) Bacterial: group A beta-haemolytic streptococcus, typhoid, mycoplasma pneumoniae
    (iii) Histoplasmosis
2. Idiopathic
3. Drugs: sulphonamides, penicillin, phenobarbitone

CAUSES OF TOXIC ERYTHEMA (a scarlet fever or measles like rash followed by peeling of the skin)

1. Infection/toxin: Group A beta-haemolytic streptococcus, staphylococcal scalded skin syndrome, toxic shock syndrome
2. Drugs
3. Kawasaki disease

FURTHER READING

Harper J 1985 Handbook of paediatric dermatology. Butterworth, Guildford
Verbov J, Morley N 1983 Colour atlas of paediatric dermatology. MTP Press, London

Infectious disease

SOME IMPORTANT INFECTIOUS DISEASES

Disease	Incubation in days	Characteristics and complications	Communicability
Chicken pox	14(7–21)	Vesicles spread down face, trunk, proximal parts of limbs. Pneumonia, ataxia	−2 to +7 days from start of rash, spots crusted (dry)
Diphtheria	3(1–6)	Grey–white membrane in nose, throat, 'toxic', myocarditis, bulbar palsy	4 weeks or negative swabs ×2
Enteric bacteria (salmonella etc, E. coli)	3–23	Three major patterns: 1. Diarrhoea 2. Septicaemia 3. Cholera like	Until asymptomatic and 3 negative stools
Fifth or slapped cheek disease	4–14	Bright red spots on cheeks, coalesce to look like a 'slap'. Fine rash to body	1 week; not apparent under 2 years old
Glandular fever (Infectious mononucleosis)	2–8 weeks	Sore throat, fever, lethargy, glands+++, hepatosplenomegaly, encephalitis, polyneuritis	3 months, avoid salivary contact (cups, kissing!)
Poliomyelitis	14(7–21)	'Cold', diarrhoea, muscle aches; after 7 days 'meningitic' and temperature rises again. Paralytic phase 3–7 days after onset of pre-paralytic meningitic phase. Spinal and bulbar forms	Until stool -ive for virus, i.e. weeks

Disease	Incubation in days	Characteristics and complications	Communicability
Roseola	10(5–15)	Fever for 3–4 days, as temperature falls rose–pink papules appear on trunk, neck, arms for a day	
Rubella	17(14–19)	Mild 'cold', then rash (fine maculopapular) which fades from face as it spreads downwards. Thrombocytopenia 3 weeks later, arthritis in adolescence, congenital infection in pregnancy	7 days from onset of rash
Infectious hepatitis	15–40	Anicteric, itchy, anorexic; to icteric, pale stools, dark urine. Tender liver/abdomen mimics appendicitis	7 days minimum
Measles	10(7–14)	'Cold', photophobia, Koplik's spots, fever, then red rash: face to trunk, conjunctivitis, otitis media, pneumonia. Encephalitis day 5–10 of illness	From 'cold' to 7 days after rash appears
Mumps	17(14–28)	Fever, sore throat, pain on chewing, furred tongue, swollen parotid. Meningoencephalitis. Rarely, orchitis, pancreatitis in children	−9 to +9 days after onset of swelling or when the swelling goes
Pertussis	10(7–14)	Catarrhal for 1–2 weeks, then paroxysmal cough ± whoop 14–100 days, recurs for up to 2 years. Death 1% <6 months old	5 weeks from onset of cough
Scarlet fever	2–5	Tonsilitis, red spots on palate, strawberry tongue, red face with circum-oral pallor, fine red rash spreads to whole of body by 2–3 days, may then shed fine skin scales. Arthritis, nephritis	3 days from start of penicillin

CAUSES OF ACUTE VIRAL RASHES

Type of rash	Likely virus
Maculopapular	Measles, rubella, coxsackie, ECHO, glandular fever (GF), cytomegalovirus
Petechial	Coxsackie, ECHO, GF (exclude meningococcaemia, scarlet fever, Henoch-Schönlein purpura, drugs, typhoid etc — see p. 129)
Telangiectatic	ECHO
Urticarial	Coxsackie, ECHO
Vesicular	Chickenpox, herpes simplex, coxsackie

CAUSES OF PYREXIA OF UNKNOWN ORIGIN (being a fever which may occur intermittently over a fortnight)

1. Infections: respiratory, urinary tract, central nervous system (e.g. tuberculosis), osteomyelitis, endocarditis, brucellosis, salmonellosis, glandular fever
2. Collagenoses: rheumatoid arthritis, lupus erythematosus
3. Malignancy: leukaemia, lymphoma, neuroblastoma, reticulum cell sarcoma
4. Miscellaneous: Crohn's, thyroiditis, diencephalic syndrome, salicylate toxicity, dehydration fever, immunodeficiency, Kawasaki disease, Munchausen by proxy

Alternative strategy (in order of frequency)
1. Viral infection: glandular fever, cytomegalovirus, viral hepatitis
2. Pneumonitis: partially treated pneumonia, mycoplasma pneumoniae, psittacosis
3. Urinary tract infection
4. Bacterial, especially gastrointestinal: typhoid, brucella, tuberculosis
5. Foreign travel: malaria, amoebiasis, typhoid, brucella, tuberculosis
6. Rare: Still's disease, subacute bacterial endocarditis, toxoplasmosis, lymphoma, Wilms' tumour

Community paediatrics

ADOPTION (CHILDREN'S ACT 1975)

The assumption of parental rights and duties, usually when one of the natural parents marries or remarries. An adopter may be married or single

Methods
1. Direct by parent with adopter
2. Third party (an intermediary) between parent and adopters. The local authority must be notified and can stop it
3. Local authority social work department
4. Registered voluntary adoption societies

CARE

Indication for a local authority to take a child into care. A child is in need of care and control which he is unlikely to get at home through:
1. Death, illness or desertion by parents
2. Neglect
3. Prevention of 'proper development' or health which happens, may happen, or has happened to this or another child in the same household
4. Exposure to moral danger
5. Beyond parental or guardian control
6. Non-attendance at school when of compulsory school age
7. Guilty of an offence other than murder. (The age of criminal responsibility is 10 years)

N.B. 1 and 2: *Children's Act*, 1948; 3–7: *Children and Young Persons Act*, 1969

Place of safety order
When care proceedings are likely or a child is about to leave the country, and he is under 17 years old, a Justice of the Peace can order him to be detained for up to 28 days in a safe place e.g. local authority or voluntary community home, police station, hospital

167

FURTHER READING

Holden A 1982 Child care legislation. In: Hart I (ed) Child care in general
  practice. Churchill Livingstone, Edinburgh, pp 29–40

NON-ACCIDENTAL INJURY (NAI)

Definition
The result of acts or omissions by parent, cohabitee or guardian.
'At risk' register is held by the local authority social work
department. It will include the following categories:
1. Physical injury
2. Administration of poisonous substances
3. Severe or persistent physical neglect
4. Non-organic failure to thrive
5. Severe neglect of behavioural or emotional development
6. Sexual abuse

Radiological features — long bones
1. Subperiosteal haemorrhages, periosteal shearing
2. Calcified old periosteal haemorrhages
3. Epiphyseal separations like bucket handles
4. Metaphyseal fragmentation which on healing looks squared off
5. Fractures at different stages of healing

Radiological features — skull (differentiating fracture from vessel markings and sutures)
1. Swelling of the overlying soft tissue
2. Straight 'hard edges', not usually branching
3. Not symmetrical
4. May 'grow'/widen over weeks

Causes of misdiagnosis of NAI
1. Accidental trauma or drug ingestion
2. Infections: impetigo ('burns'), osteomyelitis
3. Coagulation defects, thrombocytopenia
4. Osteoporosis from disuse in spina bifida, cerebral palsy
5. Normal periosteal new bone formation on X-ray
6. Vitamin deficiency: scurvy, rickets
7. Bone disorders: osteogenesis imperfecta, hypo-and
   hyperphosphatasia, Caffey's disease, osteopetrosis
8. Congenital insensitivity to pain

Aid to ageing of bruises

Colour	Age in days
Red–blue	1
Dark blue to blue–brown	1–3
Green–yellow	7–10
Yellow–brown	> 8
Fading to pink	14–28

SEXUAL ABUSE

Definition
The involvement of dependent, developmentally immature children and adolescents in sexual activities that they do not truly comprehend, that they cannot give informed consent to, or that violate the social taboos of family roles (Kempe)

Cause for suspicion from history
1. Family 'secrets'
2. Sexual knowledge, preoccupation or behaviour beyond her years
3. Sleep disturbance with nightmares, may have sexual content
4. Girl takes over mothering role whether mother present or not
5. Inappropriate, excessive displays of affection between parent and child
6. Moody, isolated, regressive behaviour
7. Medical presentation with abdominal pain, recurrent 'cystitis', perineal inflammation, discharge or vaginal bleeding

Cause for suspicion from genital examination
1. Genital injury, may be minor
2. Perineal irritation, discharge or unexplained bleeding
3. Abormal dilatation of the urethra, anus or vaginal opening
4. Foreign body inserted in a perineal orifice or in bladder
5. Purulent vaginal discharge
6. Semen present

FURTHER READING

Porter R 1984 Child sexual abuse within the family. Ciba Foundation, Tavistock Publications, London

MUNCHAUSEN'S SYNDROME BY PROXY (MEADOW'S SYNDROME)

Definition
The deliberate administration of drugs or fabrication of illness, usually by the mother, likely to lead to repeated medical investigation and treatment of a child

Common presentations
1. Neurological: convulsions, drowsiness or coma, unsteadiness
2. Blood in urine, vomit, faeces, sputum or smeared on nose or perineum
3. Rashes from rubbing, abrading the skin, applying caustics or colouring
4. Fever fabricated
5. Adulteration of urine or blood samples with chemicals etc
6. 'Allergies' (p. 136)

Causes for suspicion
1. Parent a 'Munchausen' (may not have been previously suspected), a nurse or claiming a medical relative
2. Siblings also affected, at increased risk of NAI or 'cot death'
3. The child previously severely ill in infancy

FURTHER READING

Meadow R 1984 Factitious illness — the hinterland of child abuse. In: Meadow R (ed) Recent Advances in Paediatrics 7. Churchill Livingstone, Edinburgh, pp. 217–232

CAUSES OF EDUCATIONAL DIFFICULTIES

Common
1. Emotional: lack of motivation, peer pressure, deprivation and depression
2. Neurological and sensory
   (i) Low intelligence
   (ii) Developmental disorders: dysphasia, dyslexia, dyscalculia (arithmetic difficulties)
   (iii) Deafness, especially secretory otitis media
   (iv) Visual defects: refractive error etc
3. Physical disabilities e.g. asthma, diabetes mellitus (severity not necessarily commensurate with underachievement)
4. School e.g. poor teaching, absenteeism, frequent change of school

Uncommon
1. Epilepsy e.g. petit mal
2. Drugs e.g. phenobarbitone

3. Brain injury e.g. cerebral palsy
4. Progressive dementias e.g. Batten's disease, subacute sclerosing pan encephalitis

EDUCATION ACT 1981

Implements the Warnock Report on the educational needs of all children who have 'special educational needs'. This includes not only the mentally handicapped and cerebral palsied, hearing and vision impaired, but also those with asthma, diabetes, behaviour problems etc. 'They have significantly greater difficulty in learning than the majority of children of their age, or have a disability which prevents or hinders them from making use of the educational facilities generally provided for children of their age.'

The local authority's education department has the duty to:
1. Identify all children in need, from the age of 2 years, assess their needs and review them annually until 15 years old
2. Find, as first choice, special provision in *normal* school, as long as the parents agree e.g. classroom amplification equipment for the hearing impaired, remedial teaching for specific learning difficulties
3. Ensure it is in the best interests of the child *and* his peers

The *Statement of Needs* drafted by the education department is based on assessments by many professionals (often already involved) e.g. teachers, social workers, child psychologists and psychiatrists, general practitioners and paediatricians. A copy must be given to the parents.

Parents have the right of appeal to the local authority and, ultimately, the Secretary of State for Education

CONTRAINDICATIONS TO IMMUNISATION

1. Febrile illness, intercurrent infections
2. Allergy to egg protein e.g. influenza, measles
3. 'Over immunisation' with tetanus toxoid
4. Pertussis contraindications
    (i) Previous severe local or generalised reaction (including neurological)
    (ii) Neonatal cerebral irritability or damage
    (iii) Convulsions
    Counselling indicated in:
    (i) Parent or sibling with history of idiopathic epilepsy
    (ii) Developmental delay due to neurological cause
    (iii) Neurological disease e.g. cerebral palsy
    (See latest edition of the *British National Formulary* for most recent advice)
5. No live vaccines if immuno-deficient, immuno-suppressed, on corticosteroids, leukaemic, pregnant

6. No BCG if tuberculin positive
7. Historically, no smallpox vaccine in eczema

ACTIVE IMMUNISATION

Routine Immunisation schedule

Diphtheria-pertussis-tetanus (DPT) and oral polio:

	No. Vaccinations
Start at 3–6 months	1
Repeat 4–6 weeks later	2
Then 4–6 months after second	3
School entry — omit pertussis	4
School leaving — omit pertussis and diphtheria	5

Measles: 1–2 years old

BCG: 10–13 years if Heaf test is negative

Rubella: 11–13 years for girls

Selective immunisation
1. BCG in the first week for Asian infants, or with active tuberculosis in the household
2. Hepatitis B vaccination for babies of mothers with:
    (i) Hepatitis B surface antigen (SAg) *and* hepatitis B e antigen positive with NO antibody to the e antigen
    (ii) Hepatitis B SAg positive, alone
3. Pneumococcal vaccination
    (i) Sickle cell disease
    (ii) Post-splenectomy
    (iii) Nephrotic syndrome

Some hazards of immunisation
1. Normal local or generalised reaction to TAB
2. Allergic reactions e.g. serum sickness, Arthus phenomenon, anaphylaxis, encephalitis, cyst formation
3. Provocation poliomyelitis
4. Fetal infection, damage or death from live rubella or smallpox vaccine
5. Product defects e.g. micro-organism contamination, still toxic or active
6. 'BCG-osis' in T cell immuno-deficiency
7. Kaposi eruption from smallpox vaccine
N.B. Common parental misconceptions as to contraindications include prematurity, heart disease and family history of eczema or asthma

FURTHER READING

Macfarlane J A 1984/1985/1987 Progress in child health. Vols. 1–3. Churchill Livingstone, Edinburgh
Polnay L, Hull D 1985 Community paediatrics. Churchill Livingstone, Edinburgh

Paediatric prescribing

Drug metabolism is more closely related to surface area than weight. As infants and young children have a large surface area for weight compared with adults this would result in prescribing amounts that are too small if they are just scaled down by weight e.g. a 7 kg infant might get 10% of the 70 kg adult dose. The correct dose is obtained by expressing the infant's surface area as a percentage of the adult, e.g. an average 7 kg infant is 20% of the adult surface area, i.e. twice the dose calculated by weight alone. This dose is then recommended on a weight basis of x mg/kg as the use of surface area is time-consuming and cumbersome. Further adjustment may be needed to allow for age, immaturity, organ disease etc. Paediatric dosages should not be used for adults as they may result in higher dosages than recommended.
Message: check weight and correct dosage

PHARMACOLOGICAL PROBLEMS SPECIFIC TO INFANTS AND CHILDREN

1. Immaturity of the newborn
    (i) Hepatic enzymes e.g. diazepam drowsiness, chloramphenicol toxicity in the 'grey baby syndrome'
    (ii) Renal excretion e.g. gentamycin toxicity
    (iii) Blood — Brain barrier permeability: kernicterus by displacement of bilirubin from albumin by sulphonamides etc
    (iv) Cerebral blood vessels: intraventricular haemorrhage from hyperosmolar sodium bicarbonate, especially prematures
    (v) Retinal blood vessels: oxygen toxicity? in prematures
    (vi) Haematological e.g. haemolysis from Synkavit, methaemoglobinaemia from sulphonamides, phenacetin
2. Toxic effects
    (i) Growth inhibition: corticosteroids, ACTH
    (ii) Intellectual development inhibition: antimetabolites
    (iii) Altered tissue growth: phenytoin coarsening in the face, tetracycline staining by deposition in teeth and bone

(iv) Enzyme inhibition e.g. Novobiocin inhibition of glucuronyl transferase causing hyperbilirubinaemia
3. Miscellaneous
   (i) Altered behaviour: phenobarbitone overactivity
   (ii) Tissue sensitivity e.g. increased myocardial sensitivity to digoxin in prematures

Clinical chemistry

NORMAL RANGE FOR BLOOD CONCENTRATIONS (asterisked ranges are similar to adults)

Alkaline phosphatase	35–240 U/l
Amylase	98–405 U/l*
Bicarbonate: Infancy Childhood	18–22 mmol; shl 20–26 mmol/l

Bilirubin: Total
  Infant's cord blood
 	
  2–5 days
  Childhood
  Conjugated
    Neonatal
    Childhood
	
	up to 50 μmol/l term
	up to 58 μmol/l premature
	up to 205 μmol/l
	2–14 μmol/l*
	
	up to 27 μmol/l
	0–4 μmol/l*

Calcium: First week Thereafter	1.85–2.75 mmol/l 2.20–2.76 mmol/l*
Cholesterol: Childhood	2.4–6.8 mmol/l*
Cortisol: Diurnal variation absent in first 6 weeks; thereafter p.m. value less than 50% of a.m. value	 0900 110–1076 nmol/l 2400 83–138 nmol/l
Creatine Kinase	8–60 IU/l*
Creatinine	30–80 μmol/l
Creatinine clearance: Neonates Over 1 year	40–65 ml/min/1.73 m^2 95–150 ml/min/1.73 m^3
Ferritin	10–300 μmol/l
Glucose: Up to 72 hours old,	preterm or < 2.5 kg 1.1–6.0 mmol/l term or > 2.5 kg 1.7–6.0 mmol/l

Iron:	Serum iron	14–22 μmol/l*
	Total iron binding capacity	42–66μmol/l*
Lead:	Up to	1.8 μmol/l*
Osmolality		280–300 mmol/kg*
pCO₂		4.7–6.0 kPa*
pO₂:	Newborn after 24 hours at term	9.3–13.3 kPa
	Older children	11.3–13.3 kPa*
Phosphate:	Neonates	1.20–2.78 mmol/l
	Over 1 year	1.16–1.90 mmol/l*
Potassium:	Neonate (capillary blood) up to	6.6 mmol/l
	Thereafter	3.5–5.6 mmol/l*
Protein:	Neonates total protein	46–77 g/l
	albumin	25–50 g/l
	Childhood total protein	60–78 g/l*
	albumin	35–50 g/l*
Sodium:	Neonates	130–145 mmol/l
	Thereafter	135–145 mmol/l*
Thyroid stimulating hormone: after 1st week		<5 mU/l
Thyroxine:	First week	100–400 nmol/l
	Up to 1 year	90–195 nmol/l
	Childhood	70–180 nmol/l
Transaminases		
1. Aspartate (AST)		6–17 U/l*
2. Alanine (ALT): Up to 3 months		2–27 U/l
	Thereafter	2–12 U/l*
Urea:	Infants fed cow's milk	3.3–7.5 mmol/l
	Others	2.3–6.7 mmol/l*

BIOCHEMICAL TESTS

Faecal fat
Up to 4.5 g/day on an adequate diet

Glucose tolerance test
Glucose load given decreases with increasing age and weight (2.5 g/kg to 1.25 g/kg). Normal less than 10 mmol/l at ½ and 1 hour, and less than 6.7 mmol/l at 2 hours

Growth hormone stimulation test

Normal value more than	20 mU/l
Partial deficiency	7–20 mU/l
Deficient	1–6 mU/l

D-Xylose

Give 5 g of d-xylose in 100 ml water by mouth. Normally more than 25% is excreted in the urine within 5 hours (15% if under 6 months old) or a blood concentration of more than 1.3 mmol/l at 1 hour

Urine acidification

Ammonium chloride, 5 g/1.73 m² given orally, should give a urine pH of less than 5.3 and ammonium (NH_4+) excretion of $1 \mu mol/min/1.73$ m²

FURTHER READING

Clayton B E, Jenkins P, Round J M 1980 Paediatric chemical pathology. Blackwell Publications, Oxford

Clayton B E, Round J M 1984 Chemical pathology and the sick child. Blackwell Publications, Oxford

Applying for jobs

At the present time obtaining hospital experience in paediatrics is not only an end in itself for those intent on a career in the specialty, but, for those entering General Practice in the United Kingdom, it is one of the small group of specialties essential for full accreditation. Such posts are therefore at a premium, and I make no apology for the inclusion of a chapter on job applications, in the hope that those who are unable to gain advice elsewhere will find the following guidance helpful

THE APPLICATION

The first question is, 'do you want it?' The job description obtainable from the medical staffing administrator, and a discussion with the doctor in post, will provide the relevant facts. Most hospitals have their own application forms which ask basic information.

If your handwriting is *good* you may prefer to use it, but general advice is, 'get it typed'!

No matter how many forms you have already completed, remember those selecting for interview are seeing you on paper for the first, and perhaps only, time. Make the most of your merits and accolades, avoiding the banal.

Whatever the job always give your reasons for wanting it, and why that hospital or institution.

All too often candidates fail to state what their career plans are, or declare an interest in a hospital career when applying for a General Practice training, rotating hospital post. The reverse of this particular coin is, say, when applying to academic departments within your own teaching hospital not all Professors expect their junior staff to aspire to a Chair, but check!

THE CURRICULUM VITAE (CV)

This should be properly typed. It contains details not otherwise available, and should include:
  (i) Name, age and date of birth, sex, marital status

179

(ii) a. Secondary school, appropriate distinctions such as head-boy/girl, music or sporting diplomas or awards of a higher order
   b. Intrepid experience, VSO, holiday jobs or interests with a 'caring' role or of relevance to career
(iii) University career, awards, distinctions, brief mention of unusual student attachments, projects. Extracurricular activities, Student Union, University representation in sport can be mentioned here or under leisure interests if still pursued
(iv) Final academic qualifications (not each MB), year obtained
(v) Work experience: list jobs by date, duration and content; do not be too exhaustive, a few lines suffice and should include procedures performed
(vi) Leisure pursuits: be believable and prepared to answer questions on them
(vii) Referees: always ask for their support *before* sending off the CV and inform them of the result of interview. Not only is this good manners, but failure to do either may say something about you. Before leaving this topic, remember that a prestigious referee is only as useful as the reference you are likely to receive

THE INTERVIEW

(i) The visit: this is essential. Phone the medical staffing administrator for details and ask whom to contact within the desired department. For junior posts a visit a day or two before the interview is usually sufficient, i.e. after the short list is chosen
(ii) Withdrawing: a candidate who fails to attend without notifying the committee is being discourteous, and his referees may be informed
(iii) Anticipation of questions: these will include your previous experience, publications, research, as well as your views on topics of the day of medical importance, and your future plans (however uncertain). Originality of thought is not sought, only a clear mind
(iv) The day: arrive in good time; allow twice the expected duration of travel. Dress soberly!
(v) The interview: be courteous, look at your questioner, think (not too long) before replying and be consistent, honest and to the point. Avoid arguing and getting emotional. You will be asked why you want *this* job in *this* hospital.
   At the end of the interview you may be asked if you have any questions. Do not feel obliged to ask for its own sake
Repeated failure is daunting. Ask a senior coleague for advice, but do not brood!

Preparation for the membership examination

Case histories and data interpretation: The Royal College of Physicians has now published past papers for both parts 1 and 2 at £6 and £10 respectively. In addition to supplying the answers, acceptable and non-acceptable alternative answers are listed. This should help gain insight into what the examiners require.

The clinical is divided into a long case and short cases. In the long case it is quite likely that the child has only recently been admitted with a common condition such as a febrile convulsion or asthma. The parent will probably tell you the diagnosis. The examiners know this and are likely to be more interested in your appreciation of the emotional, social, schooling and long-term implications of the condition.

The short cases are there to test your clinical examination skills. Expect to be asked to assess the development of a baby or child; know what the age-appropriate skills and milestones are and how to demonstrate them. The examiners are critical of unfamiliarity or awkwardess in using basic techniques. They expect the answer to be given in the time-honoured divisions of gross motor, fine manipulation or hand–eye coordination, speech and language, and social achievements. You may be shown a 'funny looking kid' syndrome, which even the examiner may not know the name of. Provided you are able to describe the important features you will be scoring marks. An encyclopaedic knowledge of dysmorphic conditions is not a requirement, and can even be a disadvantage.

At the oral examination you may be asked about recent experience, interesting cases, and topical items in the newspapers such as a particular case of child abuse. The well-prepared candidate will have looked at recent leading articles or review articles in the *Lancet, British Medical Journal, The New England Medical Journal*, and an authoritative paediatric journal such as *Archives of Diseases in Childhood*.

FURTHER READING

MRCP Part 1 papers
MRCP (UK) Part 2 papers
The Royal College of Physicians of London, 11 St Andrews Place, Regents Park, London NW1 4LE.

181

Glossary of syndromes

All are rare, often inherited.
(Mode: autosomal dominant = AD, autosomal recessive = AR, sex linked recessive = XL.)
Page numbers where they appear are given in brackets.

Abetalipoproteinaemia: AR ataxia, retinitis pigmentosa, thorny red cells, hypocholesterolaemia, coeliac syndrome (71, 117, 126)

Achondroplasia: AD short limb dwarfism, snub nose, frontal bossing, trident hands, occasional hydrocephalus (35, 72)

Acrodermatitis enteropathica: AR vesicular, pustular, eczematous lesions around body orifices, diarrhoea, alopecia, zinc deficiency (117, 162)

Adenosine deaminase deficiency: AR progressive severe combined immuno-deficiency (SCID), low enzyme levels in RBCs (117, 133)

Alpha-1-antitrypsin deficiency: AR prolonged obstructive neonatal jaundice, cirrhosis, adult emphysema (22, 82, 120, 121)

Alport's syndrome: hereditary glomerulonephritis with haematuria, proteinuria. Neurosensory deafness associated (144, 148)

Ataxia telangiectasia: AR progressive ataxia and choreoathetosis, pulmonary infections, telangiectasia of conjunctivae, face, elbows and knees (70, 71, 133)

Autism: see p. 63

Batten's disease: AR dementing storage disorder, blindness, fits, progressive cerebral palsy (68, 153, 171)

Beckwith's syndrome: neonatal macrosomia, macroglossia, hypoglycaemia, prominent facial naevus flameus (23, 39, 110)

Berger's disease: intermittent gross haematuria, benign focal glomerular lesion (144)

Blackfan-Diamond anaemia: congenital pure red cell hypoplasia from birth (22, 129)

Caffey's disease: infantile cortical hyperostosis of flat bones (skull, scapulae etc) and tubular bones (ulna, tibia etc) with overlying non-pitting swelling (68)

Chediak-Higashi syndrome: AR partial albinism, nystagmus, hepatosplenomegaly, lymphadenopathy, pyogenic infections, large grey — green granules in neutrophils (134)

Chronic granulomatous disease: XL frequent pyogenic infections, positive nitroblue tetrazolium test (81, 134)

Cleido-cranial dysostosis: AD absent clavicles, delayed closure of fontanelles (72)

Congenital adrenal hyperplasia: AR see p. 39

Congenital chloridorrhoea: AR newborn diarrhoea, metabolic alkalosis, low serum chloride and potassium (117)

Conn's syndrome: primary aldosteronism (102, 143, 150)

Crigler-Najjar syndrome: glucuronyl transferase deficiency, severe neonatal jaundice and AR in Type 1; milder and? AD in Type II, which responds to phenobarbitone (21, 121)

Cystic fibrosis: AR carried on chromosome 7, see p. 118

Cystinosis: AR Fanconi syndrome (146), failure to thrive, cystine crystal deposition in eyes, bone marrow, reticulo-endothelial system (148)

Dermatitis herpetiformis: vesicular, pruritic eruption; coeliac disease may be present: slow skin response to gluten free diet (162)

Diastematomyelia: boney spur through lower spinal cord, traction causing often progressive paralysis, anaesthesia, neurogenic bowel and bladder, lower limb deformities (145)

Di George's syndrome: AR defects of heart and face, neonatal tetany, repeated infections, absent thymus and parathyroids, normal immunoglobulins (117, 133, 162)

Dubin-Johnson syndrome: AR childhood intermittent obstructive jaundice, abnormal cholecystogram and bromosulphophthalein excretion, black liver pigment on biopsy (121)

Duchenne muscular dystrophy: XL often slow to walk, waddling gait, Gower's sign from 3–5 years old, pseudohypertrophy of calves, $\frac{1}{3}$ slow learners, elevated creatine phosphokinase in serum, suggestive electromyography and muscle biopsy. Half are new mutations without family history (3, 71, 157)

Dystrophia myotonica: AD infantile hypotonia, feeding difficulties, mental retardation, cataracts, myocarditis, later frontal baldness, infertility (2, 12, 19, 183)

Ebstein's anomaly: tricuspid valve set into right ventricle, large square heart shadow, abnormal ECG and rhythms (100, 102, 105)

Ehlers Danlos syndrome: AD recurrent dislocation of joints, easily scarred and elastic skin (129)

Endocardial fibroelastosis: thickening of endocardium, heart failure usually in infancy, often acute presentation, cause unknown (101, 103)

Enterokinase deficiency: steatorrhoea, failure of activation of trypsinogen to trypsin (117)

Evans syndrome: haemolytic anaemia found occasionally with idiopathic thrombocytopenia (130)

Fallot's tetralogy: infundibular obstruction, overriding aorta, ventricular septal defect, right ventricular hypertrophy (94–106)

Familial dysautonomia: see Riley-Day syndrome

Fanconi's anaemia: AR congenital malformation of forearm bones, short stature, mental retardation. Onset of pancytopenia in toddler (146)

Friedreich's ataxia: AR spinocerebellar degeneration, pes cavus, myocarditis, later scoliosis and occasionally diabetes mellitus (54, 61, 70 157)

Fröhlich's syndrome: obesity, hypogonadism, diabetes insipidus, growth failure from hypothalamic damage, usually due to tumour (43, 49)

Fructosaemia: hereditary fructose intolerance, deficient in fructose-1-phosphate aldolase, sweating, vomit, convulsions, jaundice in neonate, failure to thrive, cirrhosis and convulsions in infancy (48, 121, 142)

Galactosaemia: AR see p. 152 and pp. 22, 26, 48, 73, 121, 142, 146

Gaucher's disease: AR see p. 154 and pp. 60, 81, 130
von Gierke's disease: AR see p. 152, 159
Gilbert's syndrome: AD mild fluctuating unconjugated
  hyperbilirubinaemia, nicotinic acid administration increases jaundice (21,
  121)
Glucose-6-phosphate dehydrogenase deficiency (G-6-PD): XL dominant,
  common inborn error in Blacks, Asians, Chinese, Mediterranean stock.
  Haemolytic, Heinz body inclusions (125), crisis in neonate or later from
  drugs (127). (3, 127, 128, 134)
Glutathione synthetase deficiency: like G-6-PD
Haemolytic uraemic syndrome: acute renal failure, microangiopathic
  haemolytic anaemia, thrombocytopenia, may be preceded by shigella
  dysentery (66, 102, 116, 119, 124, 127, 130, 141, 143, 147)
Haemophilia: XL factor VIII low or absent, prolonged clotting time, normal
  bleeding time. 20% new mutations i.e. not inherited
Haemophilia B, Christmas disease: XL factor IX deficiency, differentiate
  from haemophilia by specific factor assay
Haemorrhagic shock encephalopathy syndrome: acutely ill infant,
  encephalopathy, shock, metabolic acidosis, DIC, diarrhoea +/− blood,
  renal and hepatic failure, blood ammonia rarely raised (see Reye's
  syndrome) (116, 130)
Hand-Schüller-Christian disease: triad of bone lesions, exophthalmos,
  diabetes insipidus, due to histiocytic infiltration (47)
Hartnup disease: AR generalised neutral amino aciduria, intermittent
  ataxia, photodermatitis and psychosis (71)
Hirschsprung's disease: 1 in 1000, often familial, absent ganglion cells in
  rectum, excess cholinesterase on staining biopsy section. Delay in
  passing meconium, abdominal distension, tight anus hugs examining
  finger. Obstruction, failure to thrive, diarrhoea, enterocolitis later (6, 21,
  24, 25, 35, 74, 112, 113, 116, 122)
Histidinaemia: AR see p. 153
Histiocytosis X: eosinophilic granuloma of bone, Hand-Schüller-Christian
  disease and Letterer-Siwe disease group of reticuloses (47, 81, 161)
Homocystinuria: AR see p. 153
Huntington's chorea: AD carried on chromosome 4. Neurodegeneration,
  involuntary movements, personality change, onset at 30+ years, rarely in
  childhood (2, 62, 75)
Immotile cilia syndrome: AR abnormal cilia function in respiratory tract,
  sinusitis, serous otitis media, bronchiectasis, infertility due to sperm
  immotility, situs inversus in 50% (79, 82, 83)
Incontinentia pigmenti: XL dominant, females only, linear vesicles over
  limbs, becoming warty then pigmented streaks along trunk and limbs (20,
  27)
Intestinal lymphangiectasia: protein losing enteropathy, failure to thrive,
  abdominal distension, oedema of limb(s) due to malformed lymphatics
  (117)
Jervell-Lange-Nielsen syndrome: AR familial congenital deafness, syncope,
  sudden death (101)
Kallman's syndrome: XL anosmia, gonadotrophin deficiency (43)
Kartagener's syndrome: situs inversus and immotile cilia syndrome (79, 82,
  83)
Kasabach-Merritt's syndrome: giant haemangioma, platelet trapping and
  consumption (130)

Kawasaki disease: pyrexia 5 days, conjunctivitis, red tongue, swollen hands and feet, skin peeling around nails, cervical lymphadenopathy, measles like rash. Myocarditis, coronary artery aneurysms in 10% (64, 81, 100, 101, 105, 116, 144, 163)

Lawrence-Moon-Biedl syndrome: AR retinitis pigmentosa, hypogonadism, obesity, polydactyly, mental retardation (43, 49)

Leigh's disease: AR subacute necrotising encephalopathy with progressive neurological deterioration in an infant with vomiting, dehydration and lactic acidosis (62)

Leiner's disease: severe seborrhoeic eczema, persistent diarrhoea and failure to thrive, bacterial infections, abnormal C5 complement function (134, 161)

Lesch-Nyhan syndrome: XL psychomotor deterioration in infancy, choreoathetosis and self-mutilation by 2 to 3 years old. Abdominal pain, uric acid crystaluria, renal failure, elevated plasma uric acid, absence of an enzyme (3, 142, 154, 159)

Letterer-Siwe disease: purpuric seborrhoeic eczema, hepatosplenomegaly, widespread infiltration of tissues by histiocytes in infancy (81, 120, 161)

Lowe's syndrome: XL cataract, glaucoma, Fanconi syndrome, mental retardation from infancy (73, 145, 146)

Lucey-Driscoll syndrome: familial transient unconjugated hyperbilirubinaemia due to glucuronyl transferase inhibitor in mother and baby's serum (21)

Maple syrup urine disease: AR see p. 153

Marfan syndrome: AD span greater than height, hyperextendible joints, scoliosis, lens dislocation. Dissecting aortic aneurysm in adults (32, 129, 157)

McArdle's syndrome: AR see p. 152

McCune-Albright syndrome: feathery edged pigmentation, fibrous dysplasia of bone, precocious puberty (42)

Mediterranean fever: AR repeated severe abdominal pain, chest pain, arthritis, Amyloidosis in adults (159)

Menke's kinky hair syndrome: XL depigmented curly hair, fits, psychomotor deterioration, low plasma copper and caeruloplasmin (66)

Möebius' syndrome: congenital cranial nerve nuclei agenesis, uni- or bilateral, affecting eye, face or tongue movement (58, 60)

Morquio's syndrome: AR see p. 154

Munchausen syndrome by proxy: see p. 170 (110, 116, 119, 136, 144)

Nephrogenic diabetes insipidus: XL unresponsive to antidiuretic hormone, polyuria, low urine osmolality, polydipsia, tendency to hypernatraemia, brain damage, anorexia, failure to thrive (3)

Nesidioblastosis: congenital hyperplasia of the islets of the pancreas, presenting as hypoglycaemia with hyperinsulinism in neonate or early infancy (23)

Niemann-Pick's disease: AR see p. 154 (81, 121)

Noonan's syndrome: normal chromosomes in male or female with Turner's syndrome characteristics (40, 43)

Orotic aciduria: AR megaloblastic anaemia, leucopenia, failure to thrive, crystalluria with haematuria (124)

Osteogenesis imperfecta
  Congenita: AR multiple fractures at birth, excessive sweating.
  Tarda: AD fractures in infancy, easy bruising, blue sclera, early oteosclerosis (168)

Osteopetrosis: AR thickened fragile bones, pancytopenia, splenomegaly (129, 168)

Pendred's syndrome: AR see p. 47

Pierre Robin syndrome: sporadic or familial (as part of Stickler's syndrome) cleft palate, small jaw, airway obstruction from tongue falling back into pharynx (19, 81)

Pompe's disease: AR see p. 152 (60, 71)

Potter's syndrome: see p. 19 (141)

Prader-Willi syndrome: obesity, mental retardation, hypogonadism, cryptorchid (12, 40, 49, 71)

Progeria: low birth weight, early growth failure, premature senility (72)

Pyruvate kinase: AR haemolytic disorder, inability to use glucose efficiently due to enzyme deficiency (21, 22, 126)

von Recklinghausen's disease/neurofibromatosis: AD 5+ cafe-au-lait patches 1 cm+ diameter, axillary freckles, gliomas, hypertension, later sarcomas, vertebral collapse, Schwannomas (3, 42, 61, 157, 161)

Reye's syndrome: encephalopathy, hypoglycaemia, shock, acidaemia, raised blood ammonia and serum transaminases by factor of 3 or more, diagnostic liver biopsy changes (48, 66, 69, 70, 147)

Riley-Day syndrome: AR no tears, excessive drooling, sweating, skin blotching, paroxysmal hypertension, insensitive to pain (70, 117)

Rotor syndrome: AD like Dubin-Johnson but earlier onset, no abnormal cholecystogram or liver pigment (121)

Russell-Silver syndrome: short stature, body asymmetry, triangular face, clinodactyly (32, 35, 72)

Severe combined immunodeficiency (SCID): usually AR see p. 133 (3)

Shwachman's syndrome: AR exocrine pancreatic insufficiency with normal sweat sodium, cyclical neutropenia, short stature, ichthyotic skin (125, 133)

Smith-Lemli-Opitz syndrome: AD/AR sparse hair, bulbous nose, large ears, long philtrum, thin upper lip (40)

Spasmus nutans: abnormal head posture and movements with nystagmus in infancy (158)

Spherocytosis: AD haemolytic anaemia, splenomegaly, mild jaundice, see p. 127 (22, 124, 128)

Spondylo-epiphyseal dysplasia: short trunk, mild proximal shortening of limbs, absent ossification centres of affected bones on X-ray (32)

Sotos syndrome: rapid early growth, especially skull, hands and feet, advanced bone age, mental retardation (39, 72)

Staphylococcal scalded skin syndrome: exfoliatin, a toxin usually from phage group II; erythematous, macular rash, then sheet-like separation of skin over face, trunk, limbs (163)

Stickler syndrome: AD Pierre Robin syndrome, myopia, cataracts, deafness, occasional spondylo-epiphyseal dysplasia (see Pierre Robin syndrome)

Sturge–Weber anomaly: port wine stain, ophthalmic division of 5th cranial nerve, ipsilateral intracranial calcification, glaucoma, focal seizures, hemiplegia, mental retardation (73)

Subacute sclerosing panencephalitis: progressive dementia, spasticity, fits with burst-suppression pattern on EEG, measles antibody in CSF (62, 66, 68, 171)

Tay-Sachs disease: AR see p. 154 (68)

Testicular feminisation: XY chromosomes, external genitalia female, absent menarche and often sexual hair. Cells do not respond to androgens (40, 43)

TORCH: congenital infections; toxoplasmosis, other e.g. syphilis, AIDS, rubella, cytomegalovirus, herpes simplex (2, 16, 65, 66)

Toxic shock syndrome: staphylococcal toxin, usually menstruating using tampon, scarlatiniform rash, 'gastroenteritis', fever, conjunctivitis, pharyngitis, shock; later skin peels (116, 163)

Tuberous sclerosis: AD epilepsy, white leaf shaped macules in infancy, facial adenoma sebaceum from school age, mental retardation, subependymal nodules in brain CT scan (20, 27, 42, 61, 65, 67, 145)

Tyrosinosis: tyrosine in urine (121)

Tyrosinaemia: AR see p. 153

Vitamin D resistant rickets: XL dominant, rickets in older infant or child needing huge doses of vitamin D and phosphate supplements (3, 151)

von Willebrand's disease: AD prolonged bleeding time due to low factor VIII related antigen (renamed von Willebrand factor) consequent reduced factor VIII and platelet adhesion (44, 130, 131)

Werdnig-Hoffman disease: AR hypotonia, muscle fibrillation, early infancy or toddler types. Electromyograph characteristic of anterior horn cell degeneration (3, 71)

William's syndrome: facies, mental retardation, supravalvular aortic stenosis, raised blood pressure, bone changes± hypercalcaemia (96, 151)

Wilson's disease: AR jaundice, hepatosplenomegaly, occasionally haemolytic anaemia; low serum caeruloplasmin, increased hepatic copper. Neurological deterioration and Fanconi's syndrome may occur in child (62, 75, 120, 121, 146, 148)

Wilson-Mikity syndrome: prematures get severe respiratory failure for no apparent reason. Chest X-ray shows combined segmented collapse and over inflation (84)

Wiskott-Aldrich syndrome: XL thrombocytopenia, eczema, repeated infections, low IgM (3, 117, 133, 161)

Wolman's disease: AR infantile malabsorption, hepatosplenomegaly, adrenal calcification, leucocyte acid lipase absent (117, 120, 121)

Zollinger-Ellison syndrome: peptic ulceration, gastric mucosa hypertrophy and excessive acid secretion due to non-beta islet cell adenoma (117, 119)

Index